Everyday Air Fryer meals

A collection of Easy Air Fryer Recipes for Beginners

By Samantha Hendrick

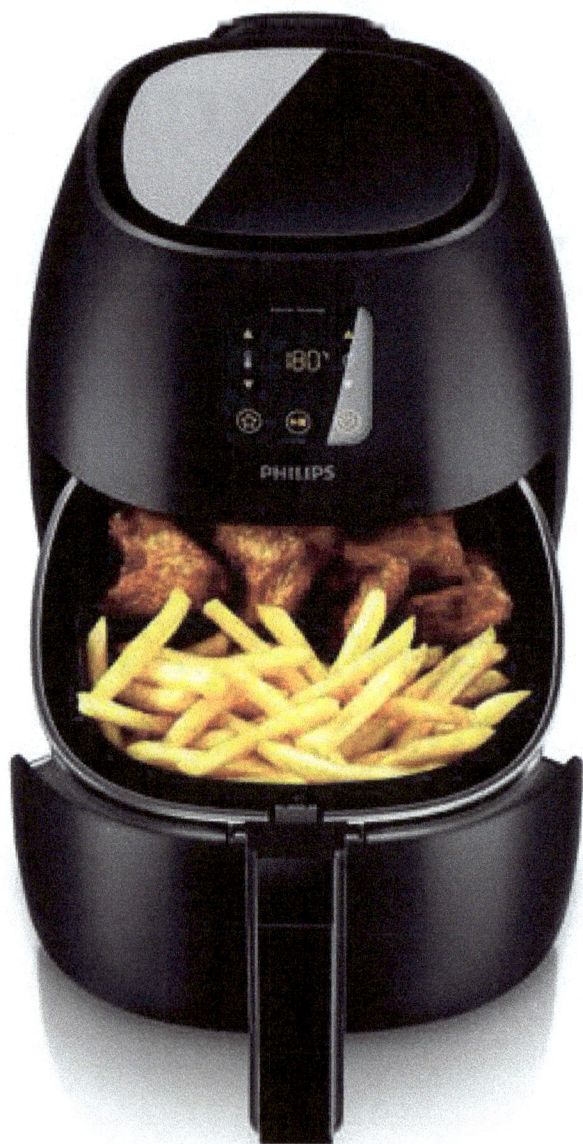

The content within this book has been derived from various sources. Please consult a licensed professional before attempting any techniques outlined in this book.

By reading this document, the reader agrees that under no circumstances is the author responsible for any losses, direct or indirect, which are incurred as a result of the use of information contained within this document, including, but not limited to, — errors, omissions, or inaccuracies.

Table of Contents

Kashmiri Chili Powder 'n Garlic Shrimp BBQ

Servings per Recipe: 4

Cooking Time: 10

Ingredients:

- 1 fresh red Chile (like Fresno), seeds removed, finely grated
- 1 tablespoon coarsely ground pepper /15g
- 1 tablespoon fresh lime juice /15ml
- 1-pound large shrimp, peeled, deveined /450g
- 2 tablespoons vegetable oil, plus more for the grill /30ml
- 3 garlic cloves, finely grated
- Kosher salt
- Lime wedges and Kashmiri chili powder or paprika (for serving)

Instructions:

1) In a large bowl, combine oil, lime juice, pepper, garlic, and Chile. Add the shrimp season with salt and let it marinate for 10 minutes.
2) Thread shrimp into steel skewers.
3) Place on skewer rack in the air fryer.
4) Cook for 5 minutes at 3900 F or 199°C .

5) Dress in chili powder, lime wedges and serve.

Nutrition Information:

- Calories per Serving: 144
- Carbs: 2.2g
- Protein: 15.6g
- Fat: 8.0g

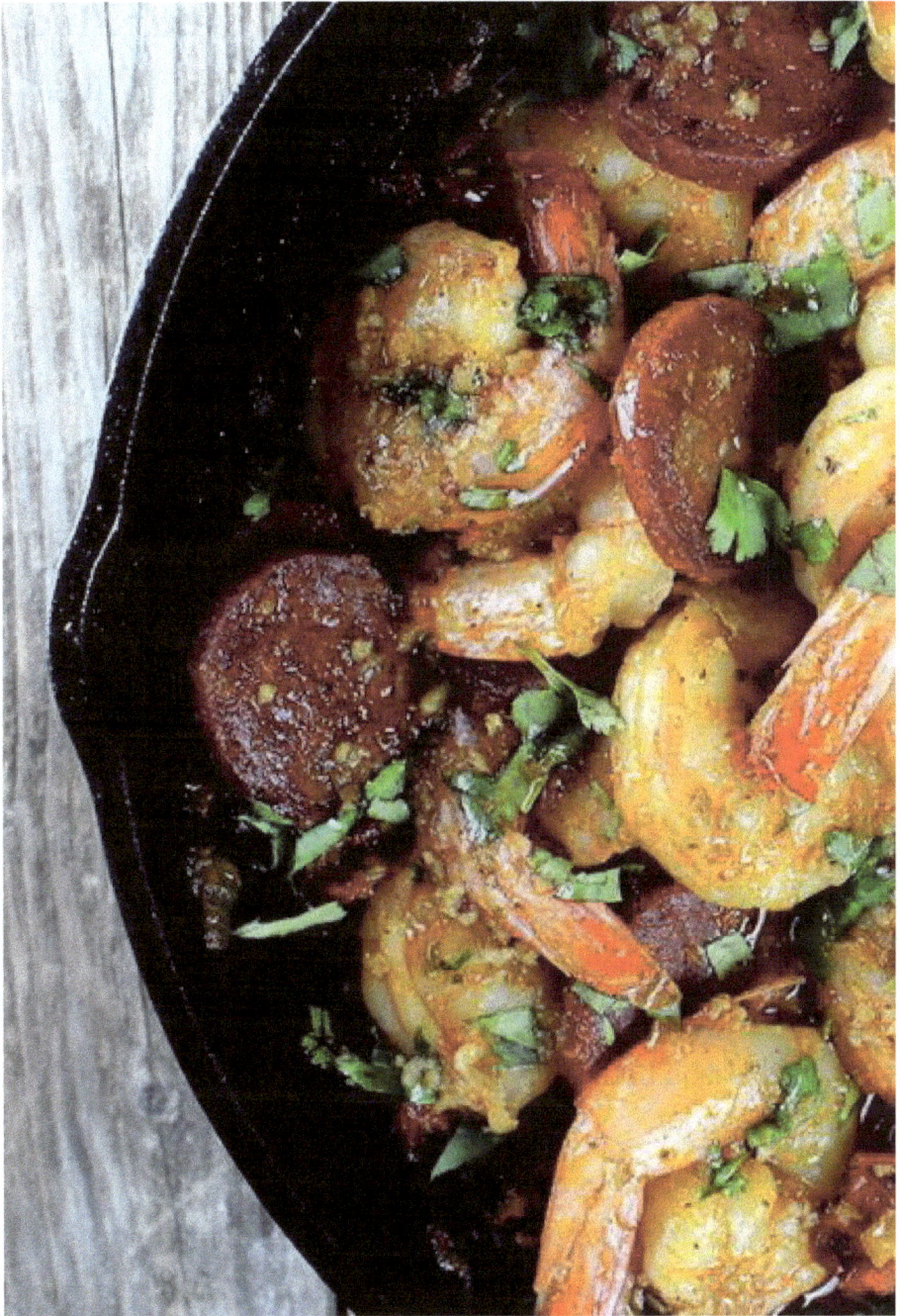

Lemony-Parsley Linguine with Grilled Tuna

Servings per Recipe: 2

Cooking Time: 20 Minutes

Ingredients:

- 1 tablespoon capers, chopped /15g
- 1 tablespoon organic olive oil /15ml
- 12 ounces linguine, cooked based on package Instructions /360g
- 1-pound fresh tuna fillets /450g
- 2 cups parsley leaves, chopped /260g
- Juice from 1 lemon
- Salt and pepper to taste

Instructions:

1) Preheat the air fryer to 3900 F or 199°C .
2) Place the grill pan in the air fryer.
3) Season both sides of the tuna with salt and pepper. polish with oil.
4) Grill for 20 minutes.
5) Shred cooked tuna into pieces using a fork and serve with cooked linguine. Sprinkle parsley and capers. Season with

salt and pepper to taste and sprinkle with freshly squeezed lemon juice.

Nutrition information:

- Calories per serving: 520
- Carbs: 60.6g
- Protein: 47.7g
- Fat: 9.6g

Lemon-Basil on Cod Filet

Servings per Recipe: 4

Cooking Time: 15

Ingredients:

- ¼ cup essential olive oil /62.5ML
- 4 cod fillets
- A lot of basil, torn
- Juice from 1 lemon, freshly squeezed
- Salt and pepper to taste

Instructions:

1) Warm air fryer for 5 minutes.
2) Season the cod fillets with salt and pepper to taste. Place in a sparingly greased baking pan.
3) Mix the remainder of the ingredients inside a bowl and stir to combine well. Pour over the fish.
4) Cook for 15 minutes at 330° F or 166°C .
5) Serve and enjoy.

Nutrition information:

- Calories per serving: 235
- Cars: 1.9g
- Protein: 14.3g
- Fat: 18.9g

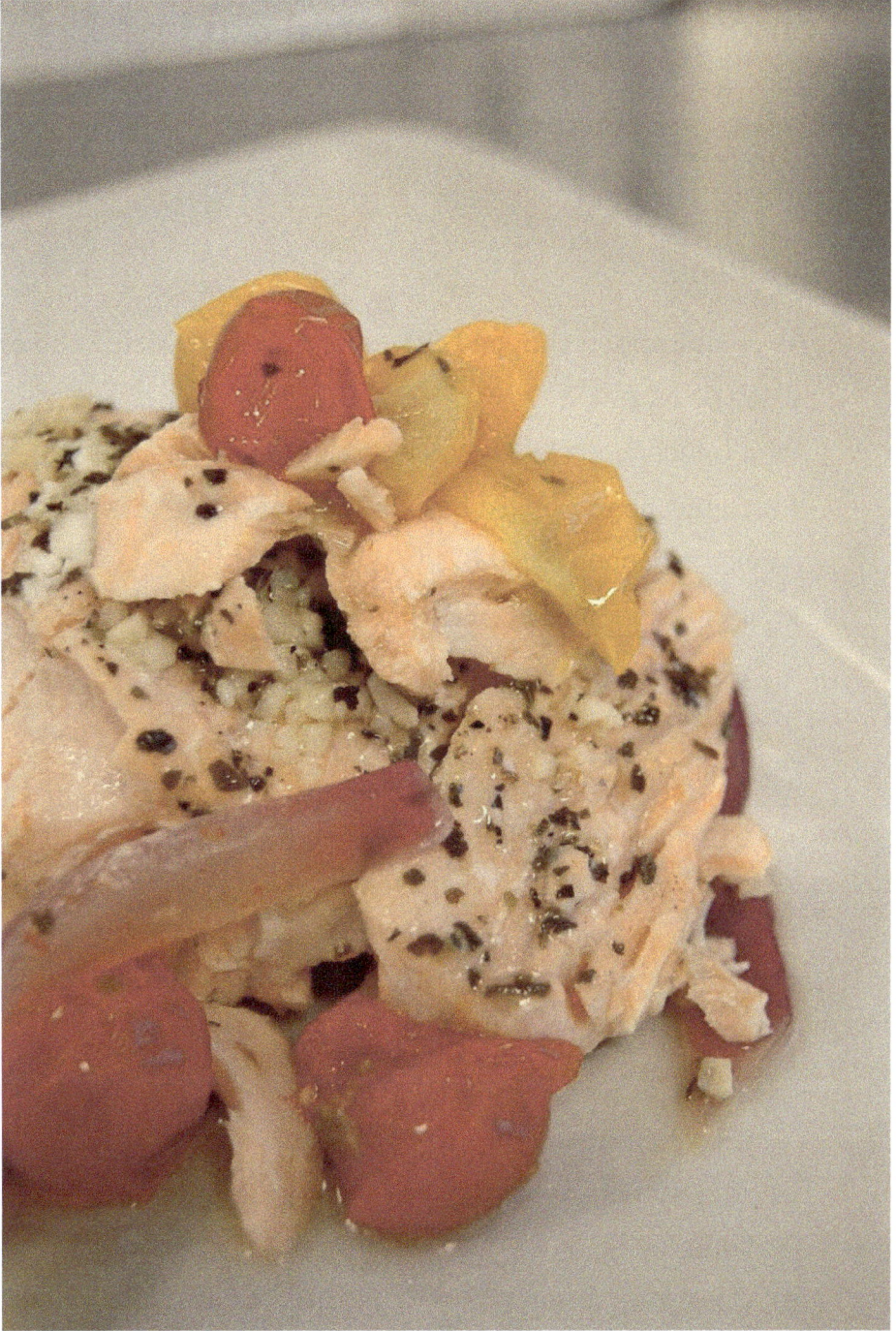

Lemon-Garlic on Buttered Shrimp Fry

Servings per Recipe: 4

Cooking Time: 15

Ingredients:

- 1 tablespoon chopped chives or 1 teaspoon dried chives /15G OR /5G
- 1 tablespoon freshly squeezed lemon juice /15ML
- 1tablespoon minced basil leaves plus more for sprinkling or 1 teaspoon dried basil /15G
- 1 tablespoon minced garlic /15G
- 1-lb defrosted shrimp (21-25 count) /450G
- 2 tablespoons chicken stock (or white wine) /30ML
- 2 teaspoons red pepper flakes /10G
- 4 tablespoons butter /60G

Instructions

1) Lightly grease the baking dish with cooking spray using any oil of your choice. Melt the butter for two minutes at 330°F or 166°C. Add red pepper flakes and garlic. Cook for 3 minutes.
2) Add remaining ingredients to a pan and Stir well to coat completely.
3) Cook for 5 minutes at 330°F or 166°C . Stir and allow it to cook for another 5 minutes.

4) Serve and enjoy

Nutrition Information:

- Calories per Serving: 213
- Carbs: 1.0g
- Protein: 23.0g
- Fat: 13.0g

Lemon-Paprika Salmon Filet

Servings per Recipe: 2

Cooking Time: 15

Ingredients:

- 1 tablespoon butter, melted /15ML
- 1 tablespoon minced fresh thyme or 1 teaspoon dried thyme /15G
- 1 teaspoon grated lemon zest /5G
- 1/2 teaspoon salt /2.5G
- 1/4 teaspoon lemon-pepper seasoning /1.25G
- 1/4 teaspoon paprika /1.25
- 1-1/2 cups soft bread crumbs /195G
- 2 garlic cloves, minced
- 2 salmon fillets (6 ounces or /180G each)
- 2 tablespoons minced fresh parsley /30G

Instructions

1) Add bread crumbs, fresh parsley thyme, garlic, lemon zest, salt, lemon-pepper seasoning, and paprika in a medium-sized bowl. Stir to combine well.
2) Lightly grease the baking dish with oil. Add salmon filet with the skin facing down. Evenly sprinkle bread crumbs on top of the salmon.

3) Cook for 10 minutes at 390°F or 199°C . Allow to sit for 5 minutes.

4) Serve and Enjoy

Nutrition Information:

- Calories per Serving: 331
- Carbs: 9.0g
- Protein: 31.0g
- Fat: 19.0g

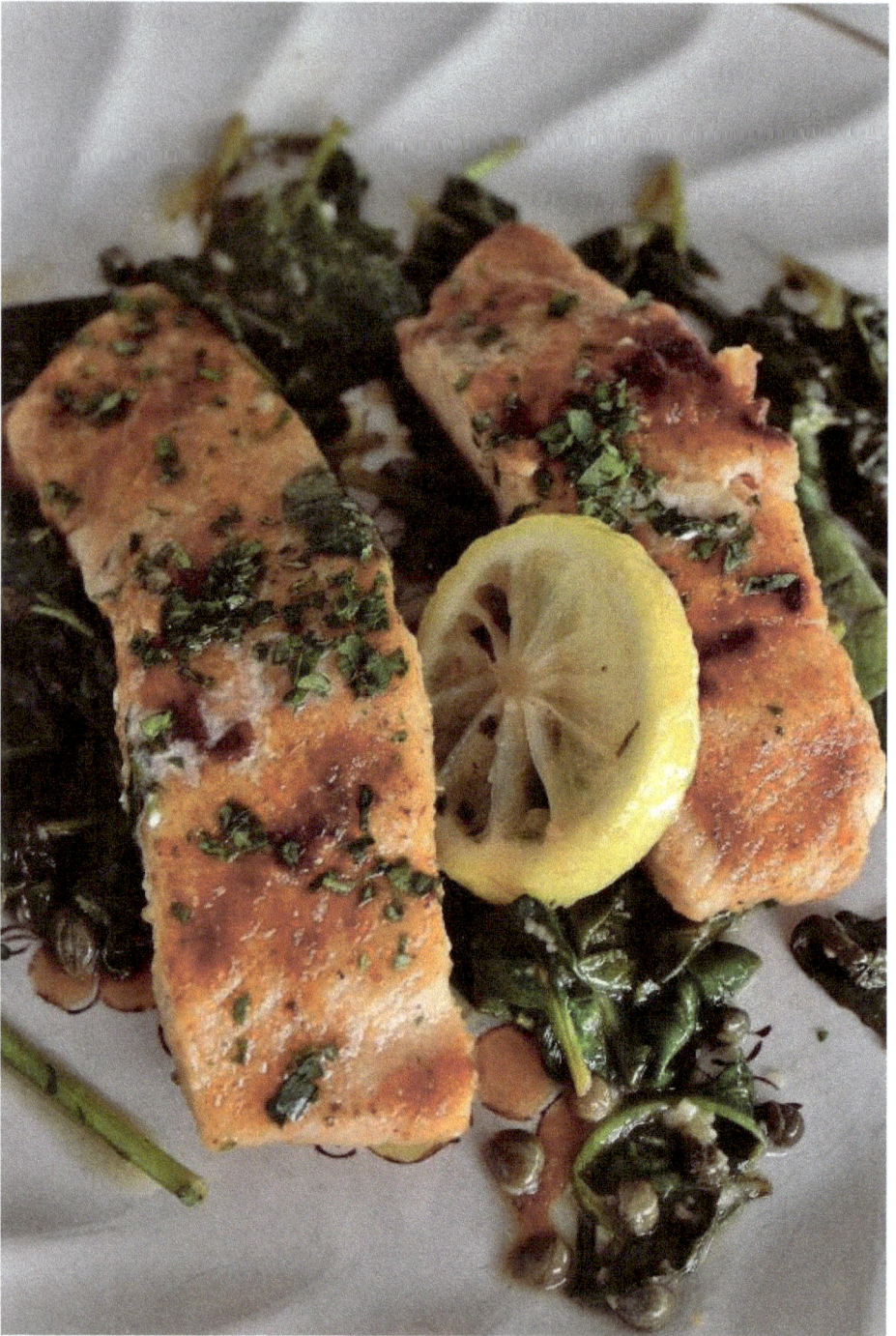

Lemon-Pepper Red Mullet Fry

Servings per Recipe: 4

Cooking Time: 15

Ingredients:

- 1 tablespoon olive oil /15ML
- 4 whole red mullets, gutted and scales removed
- Juice from 1 lemon
- Salt and pepper to taste

Instructions:

1) Preheat the air fryer to 390° F or 199°C .
2) Place the grill pan in the air fryer.
3) Season the red mullet with salt, pepper, and lemon juice.
4) Brush with extra virgin olive oil.
5) Grill for 15 minutes per batch.

Nutrition information:

- Calories per serving: 152
- Carbs: 0.9g
- Protein: 23.1g
- Fat: 6.2g

Lemony Grilled Halibut 'n Tomatoes

Servings per Recipe: 4

Cooking Time: 15

Ingredients:

- ½ cup hearts of palm, rinse and drained /65G
- 1 cup cherry tomatoes /130
- 2 tablespoons oil /30ML
- 4 halibut fillets
- Juice from 1 lemon
- Salt and pepper to taste

Instructions:

1) Preheat the air fryer to 390° F or 199°C .
2) Place the grill pan in the air fryer.
3) Season the halibut fillets with lemon juice, salt and pepper to taste. Brush with your preferred oil.
4) Place the fish in the grill pan.
5) Arrange the hearts of palms and cherry tomatoes on the side and sprinkle with more salt and pepper.
6) Allow cooking for 15 minutes.

Nutrition information:

- Calories per serving: 208
- Carbs: 7g

- Protein: 21 g
- Fat: 11g

Lemony Tuna-Parsley Patties

Servings per Recipe: 4

Cooking Time: 10 Minutes

Ingredients

- ½ cup panko bread crumbs /65G
- 1 egg, beaten
- 1 tablespoon freshly squeezed lemon juice /15ML
- 2 cans of tuna in brine
- 2 tablespoons chopped parsley /30G
- 2 teaspoons Dijon mustard /30G
- 3 tablespoons extra virgin olive oil /45ML
- A drizzle of Tabasco sauce

Instructions:

1) Remove the liquid from the canned tuna and set it in the bowl.
2) Shred the tuna in a bowl and season with mustard, bread crumbs, fresh lemon juice, and parsley.
3) Add the egg and Tabasco sauce to the mix. Stir until well combined.
4) Form shaped lumps using your hands and place them inside the fried setting for about 120 minutes.
5) Preheat mid-air fryer to 390° F or 199°C .
6) Place the grill pan in the air fryer.

7) Brush all sides of the patties with essential olive oil, place in the grill pan.

8) Cook for 10 minutes. Turn over the patties after 5 minutes for even browning.

Nutrition information:

- Calories per serving: 209
- Carbs: 2.9g
- Protein: 18.8g
- Fat: 13.5g

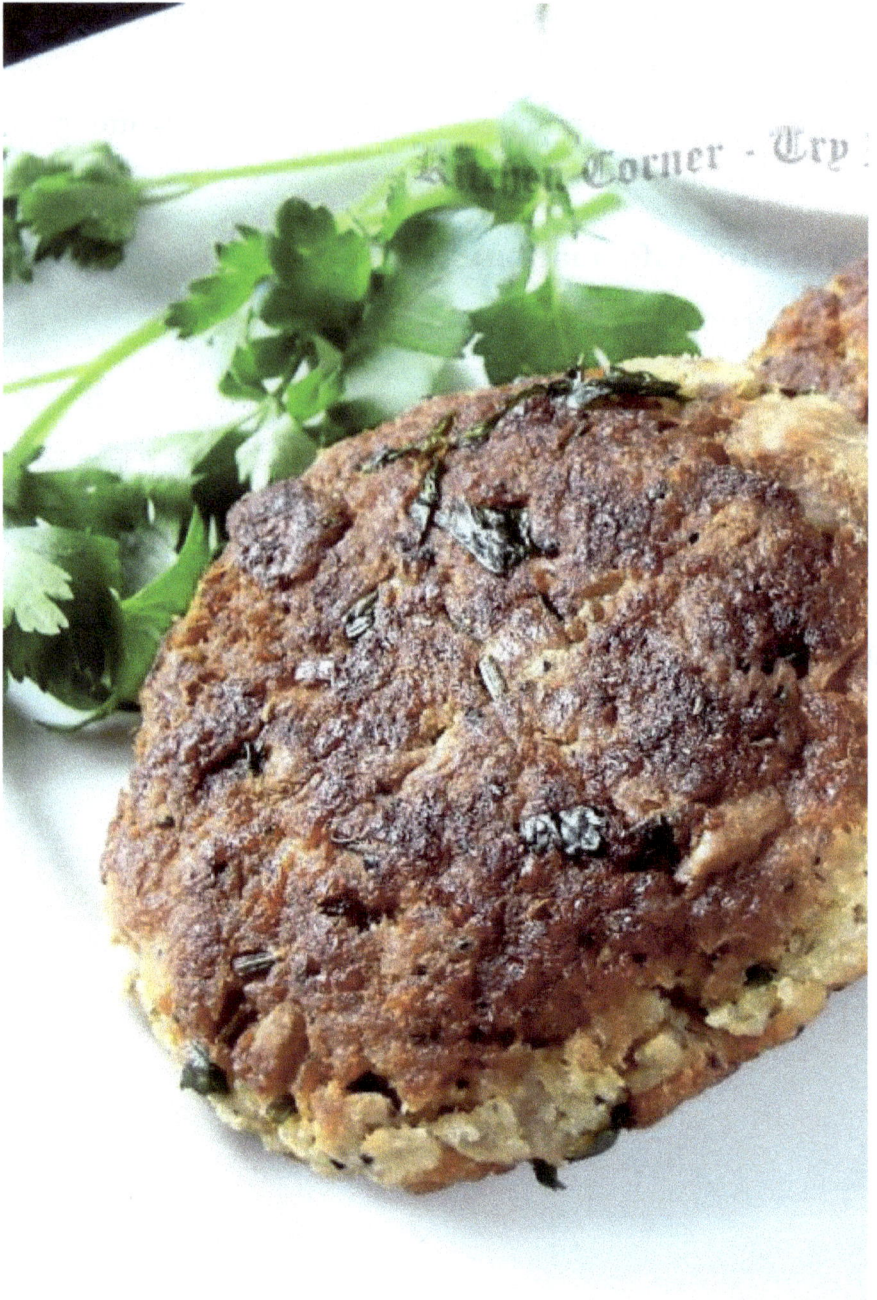

Air Fried Cod with Basil Vinaigrette

Serves: 4

Cooking Time: 15 minutes

Ingredients:

- ¼ cup olive oil /62.5ml

- 4 cod fillets

- A bunch of basil, torn

- Juice from 1 lemon, freshly squeezed

- Salt and pepper to taste

Instructions:

1) Warm up the air fryer for 5 minutes.

2) Sprinkle salt and pepper on the cod fillets.

3) Place in the air fryer and allow to cook for 15 at 3500 F or 177°C.

4) meanwhile, mix the other ingredients in a bowl and mix well to combine.

5) Serve the air fried cod using the basil vinaigrette.

Nutrition information:

- Calories per serving: 235

- Carbohydrates: 1.9g

- Protein: 14.3g

- Fat: 18.9g

Almond Flour Coated Crispy Shrimps

Serves: 4

Cooking Time: 10 minutes

Ingredients:

- ½ cup almond flour /32.5g

- 1 tablespoon yellow mustard /15g

- 1-pound raw shrimps, peeled and deveined //450g

- 3 tablespoons olive oil /45ml

- Salt and pepper to taste

Instructions:

1) Place all ingredients in a Ziploc bag and shake vigorously to combine well.

2) Place the combined ingredients in a mid-air fryer and cook for 10 Minutes at 400°F or 205°C .

Nutrition information:

- Calories per serving: 206

- Carbohydrates: 1.3g

- Protein: 23.5g

- Fat: 11.9g

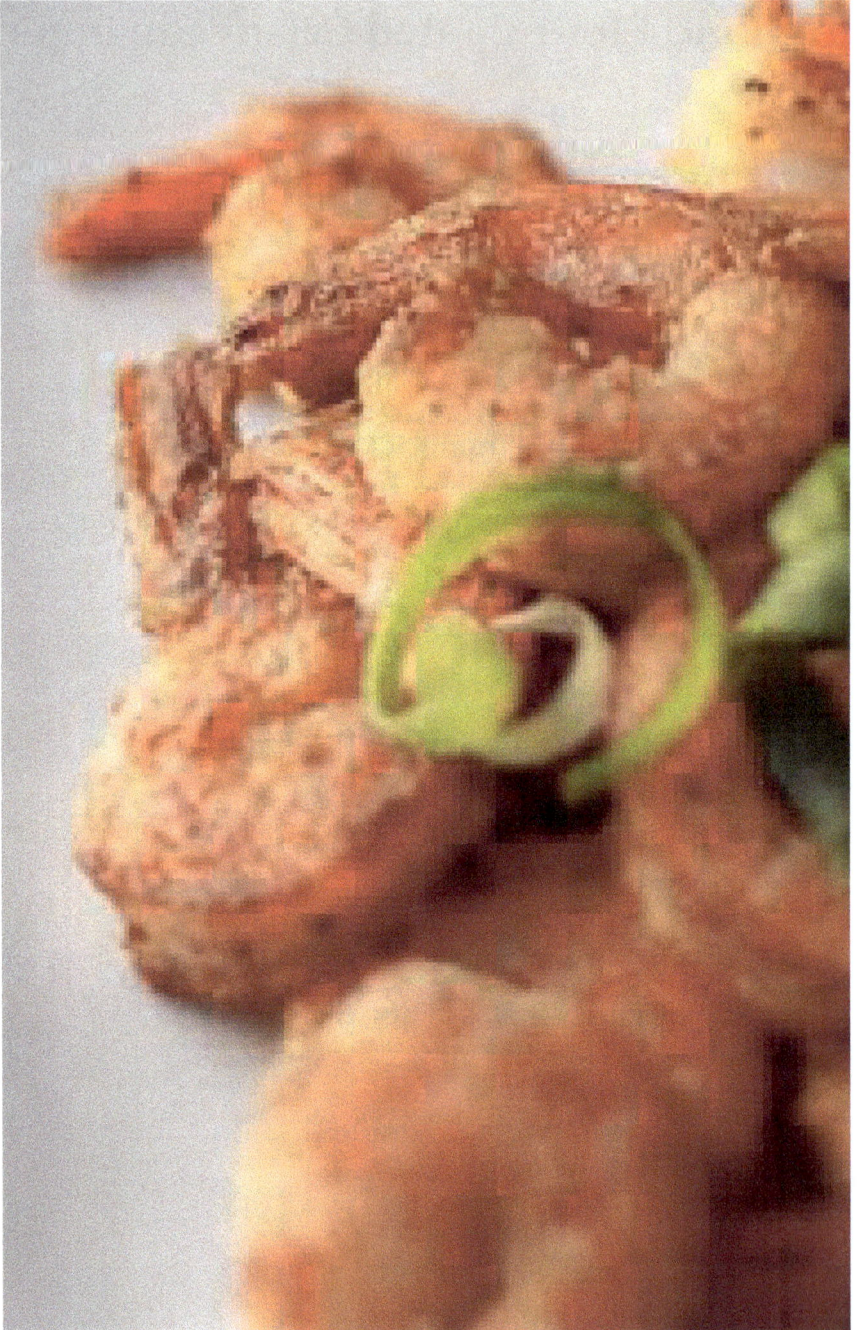

Another Crispy Coconut Shrimp Recipe

Servings per Recipe: 4

Cooking Time: 20

Ingredients:

- ½ cup flour /65g

- ½ stick cold butter, cut into cubes

- ½ tablespoon fresh lemon juice /7.5ml

- 1 egg yolk, beaten

- 1 green onion, chopped

- 1-pound salmon fillets, cut into small cubes /450g

- 3 tablespoons whipping cream /45ml

- 4 eggs, beaten

Salt and pepper to taste

Instructions:

1) Preheat your air fryer to 3900 F or 199°C.

2) Spice salmon fillets with lemon juice, salt and pepper to taste.

3) Mix the flour and butter in a bowl. Add cold water gradually while stirring to form a dough. Knead the dough into a sheet on a flat surface.

4) Place the dough in a baking pan, press the dough firmly in the baking pan.

5) Properly whisk the eggs and egg yolk in a bowl and season with salt and pepper to taste.

6) Place the salmon cubes on the baking pan lined with the dough and pour the whisked egg over it.

7) Cook for 15 to 20 minutes.

8) Dress with green onions once cooked.

Nutrition information:

- Calories per serving: 483

- Carbs: 5.2g

- Protein: 45.2g

- Fat: 31.2g

Apple Slaw Topped Alaskan Cod Filet

Servings per Recipe: 3

Cooking Time: 15

Ingredients:

- ¼ cup mayonnaise /62.5ml

- ½ red onion, diced

- 1 ½ pounds frozen Alaskan cod /675g

- 1 box wheat grains panko bread crumbs

- 1 granny smith apple, julienned

- 1 tablespoon vegetable oil /15ml

- 1 teaspoon paprika /5g

- 2 cups Napa cabbage, shredded /260g

Salt and pepper to taste

Instructions:

1) Preheat the air fryer to 3900 F or 199°C .

2) Place the grill pan accessory in the air fryer.

3) Brush some oil on the fish and place the fish in a bowl of breadcrumbs. Properly coat fish with breadcrumbs.

4) Place the fish in the grill pan and cook for seven and a half minutes, flip the fish and cook for an additional seven and a half minutes.

5) Meanwhile, prepare the slaw by mixing the residual Ingredients in the bowl.

6) Serve the fish with the slaw.

Nutrition information:

- Calories per serving: 316

- Carbs: 13.5g

- Protein: 37.8g

- Fat: 12.2g

Baked Cod Fillet Recipe From Thailand

Serves: 4

Cooking Time: 20 minutes

Ingredients:

- ¼ cup coconut milk, freshly squeezed /62.5ml

- 1 tablespoon lime juice, freshly squeezed /15ml

- 1-pound cod fillet, cut into bite-sized pieces /450g

- Salt and pepper to taste

Instructions:

1) Warm up your mid-air fryer for 5 minutes.

2) Place all ingredients in a baking pan.

3) Place the baking pan in the mid-air fryer.

4) Let it cook for 20 minutes at 3250 F or 163°C.

Nutrition information:

- Calories per serving: 844

- Carbohydrates: 2.3g

- Protein: 21.6g

- Fat: 83.1g

Brown Rice, Spinach 'n Tofu Frittata

Serves: 4

Cooking Time: 55 minutes

Ingredients:

- ½ cup baby spinach, chopped /65G
- ½ cup kale, chopped /65G
- ½ onion, chopped
- ½ teaspoon turmeric /2.5G
- 1 ¾ cups brown rice, cooked /218G
- 1 flax egg (1 tablespoon or 15G flaxseed meal + 3 tablespoons or 45ML cold water)
- 1 package firm tofu
- 1 tablespoon organic olive oil /15ML
- 1 yellow pepper, chopped
- 2 tablespoons soy sauce /30ML
- 2 teaspoons arrowroot powder /10G
- 2 teaspoons Dijon mustard /10G
- 2/3 cup almond milk /167ML
- 3 big mushrooms, chopped
- 3 tablespoons nutritional yeast /45G
- 4 cloves garlic, crushed
- 4 spring onions, chopped
- a few basil leaves, chopped

Instructions:

1) Preheat the air fryer to 375° F or 191°C . Grease a skillet with oil.

2) To prepare the frittata crust mix the brown rice and flax egg together. Flatten the rice to the baking pan and a rice crust will be formed. Polish the crust with oil and cook for 10 minutes.

3) Heat extra virgin olive oil in another skillet over medium heat and sauté the garlic and onions for 2 minutes.

4) Add the pepper and mushroom and continue stirring for 3 minutes.

5) Add kale, spinach, spring onions, and basil while stirring. Scoop the content from the pan and set it aside.

6) Add the tofu, mustard, turmeric, soy sauce, nutritional yeast, vegan milk and arrowroot powder in a blender and blend to smooth. Pour the content in a mixing bowl, add sautéed vegetables and stir.

7) Pour the vegan frittata mixture into the rice crust and cook in the air fryer for 40 minutes.

Nutrition information:

- Calories per serving: 226
- Carbohydrates: 30.44g
- Protein: 10.69g
- Fat: 8.05g

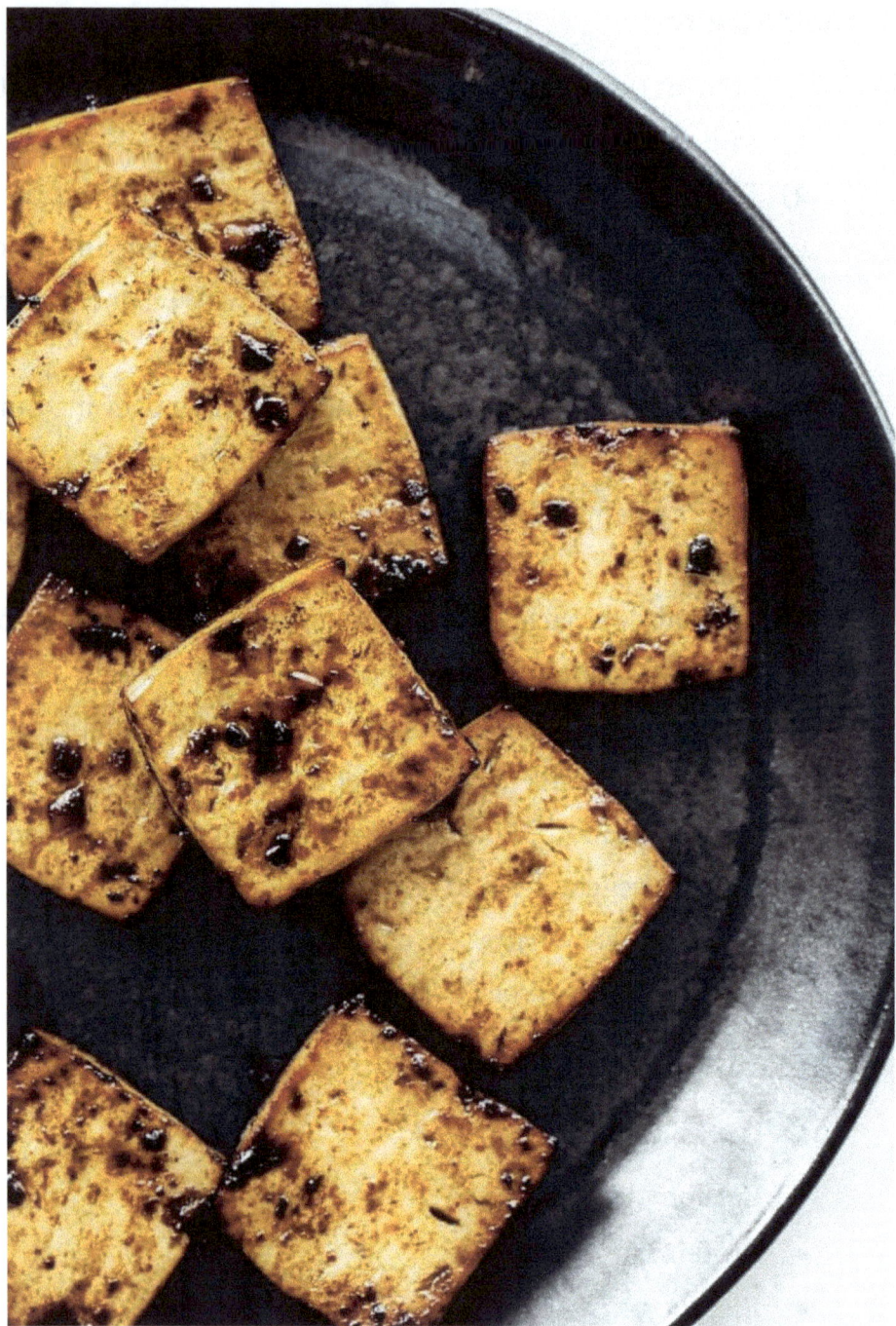

Brussels sprouts with Balsamic Oil

Serves: 4

Cooking Time: 15

Ingredients:

- ¼ teaspoon salt /1.25G
- 1 tablespoon balsamic vinegar /15ML
- 2 cups Brussels sprouts, halved /260G
- 2 tablespoons essential olive oil /30ML

Instructions:

1) Put on the air fryer and preheat for 5 minutes.
2) Grab a bowl, put all the ingredients in it and mix well to coat the zucchini fries.
3) Place the bowl in the mid-air fryer basket.
4) Allow to cook at 350° F or 177°C for 15 minutes.

Nutrition information:

- Calories per serving: 82
- Carbohydrates: 4.6g
- Protein: 1.5g
- Fat: 6.8g

Buttered Carrot-Zucchini with Mayo

Servings per Recipe: 4

Cooking Time: 25 minutes

Ingredients:

- 1 tablespoon grated onion /15G
- 2 tablespoons butter, melted /30ML
- 1/2-pound carrots, sliced /225G
- 1-1/2 zucchinis, sliced
- 1/4 cup water /62.5ML
- 1/4 cup mayonnaise /62.5ML
- 1/4 teaspoon prepared horseradish /1.25G
- 1/4 teaspoon salt /1.25G
- 1/4 teaspoon ground black pepper /1.25G
- 1/4 cup Italian bread crumbs /32.5G

Instructions

1) Grease the baking pan lightly with oil. Add carrots and allow to cook at 360° F or 183°C for 8 minutes. Add zucchini and continue cooking for another 5 minutes.

2) Add pepper, salt, horseradish, onion, mayonnaise, and water in a bowl and mix well. Pour this content into the pan containing the veggies. Mix well to coat.

3) In another bowl mix melted butter and bread crumbs. Sprinkle over veggies.

4) Cook for 10 at 390° F or 199°C until the toppings are lightly browned.

5) Serve and enjoy.

Nutrition Information:

- Calories per Serving: 223
- Carbs: 13.8g
- Protein: 2.7g
- Fat: 17.4g

Cauliflower Steak with Thick Sauce

Serves: 2

Cooking Time: 15

Ingredients:

- ¼ cup almond milk /62.5ML
- ¼ teaspoon vegetable stock powder /1.25G
- 1 cauliflower, sliced into two
- 1 tablespoon olive oil /15ML
- 2 tablespoons onion, chopped /30G
- Salt and pepper to taste

Instructions:

1) Brine or soak cauliflower in salted water for around 2 hours while preheating the air fryer to 400° F or 205°C .
2) Rinse the salt off the cauliflower, place in the air fryer and cook for 15 minutes.
3) Heat oil in a frying pan over medium heat. Sauté the onions and stir until tender. Sprinkle vegetable stock powder and milk.
4) Allow to boil and reduce heat to low.
5) Allow the sauce to cook well and season with salt and pepper.
6) Serve cauliflower steak on a plate and pour the sauce on it.

Nutrition information:

- Calories per serving: 91
- Carbohydrates:6.58 g
- Protein: 1.02g
- Fat: 7.22g

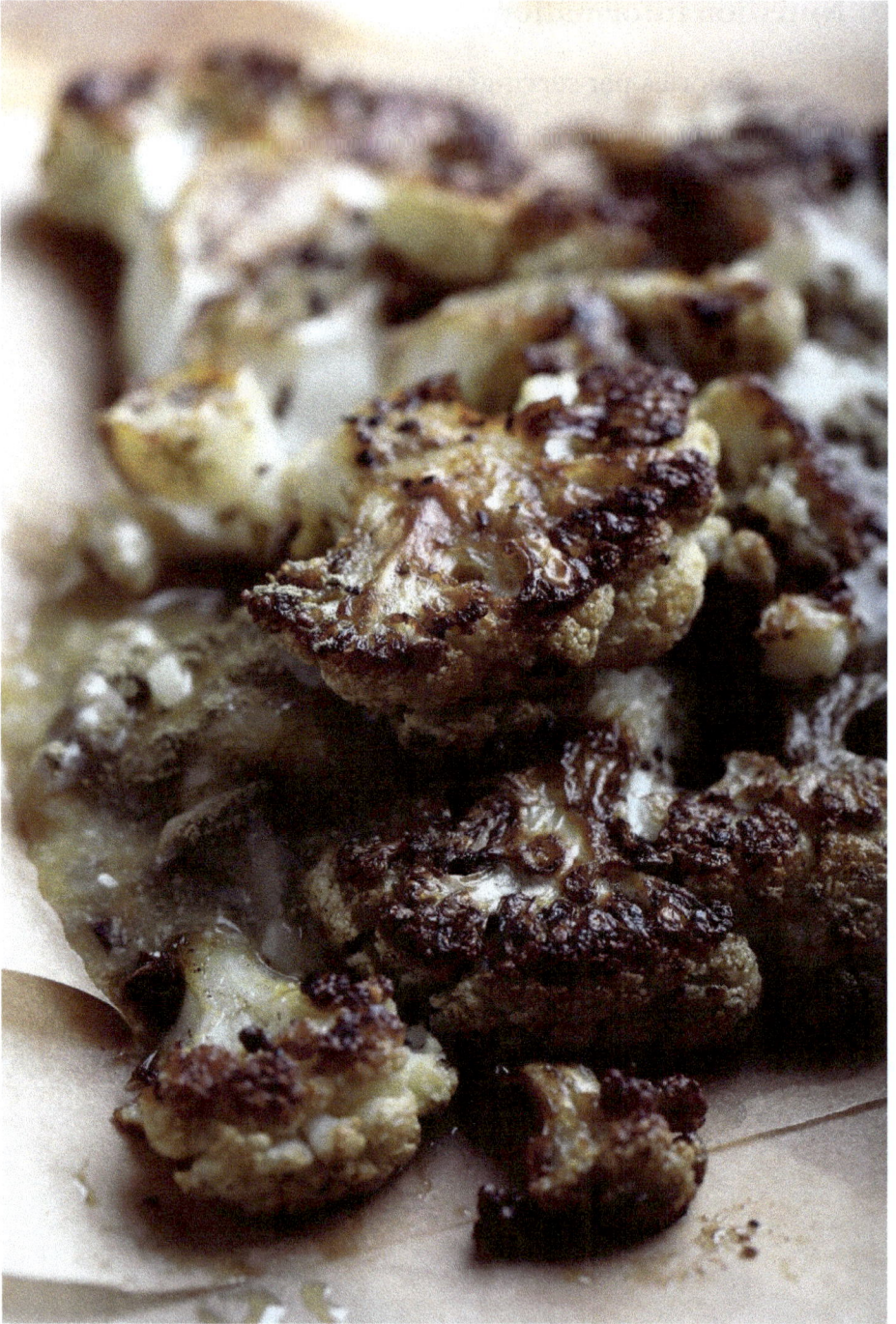

Cheddar, Squash 'n Zucchini Casserole

Servings per Recipe: 4

Cooking Time: 30 Minutes

Ingredients:

- 1 egg
- 5 saltine crackers, or when needed, crushed
- 2 tablespoons bread crumbs /30G
- 1/2-pound yellow squash, sliced /225G
- 1/2-pound zucchini, sliced /225G
- 1/2 cup shredded Cheddar cheese /65G
- 1/2 teaspoon salt /2.5G
- 1/4 onion, diced
- 1/4 cup biscuit baking mix /32.5G
- 1/4 cup butter /32.5G

Instructions

1) Grease a baking pan that fits into your air fryer lightly with cooking spray. Add onion, zucchini, and yellow squash. Cover pan with foil and cook for 15 minutes at 360° F or 183°C or until tender.

2) Add salt, sugar, egg, butter, baking mix, and cheddar cheese. Mix well. Fold in crushed crackers. Top with bread crumbs.

3) Cook for 15 minutes at 390° F or 199°C until tops are lightly browned.

4) Dish out and enjoy.

Nutrition Information:

- Calories per Serving: 285
- Carbs: 16.4g
- Protein: 8.6g
- Fat: 20.5g

Mushroom 'n Bell Pepper Pizza

Serves: 10

Cooking Time: 10 Minutes

Ingredients:

- ¼ red bell pepper, chopped
- 1 cup oyster mushrooms, chopped /130G
- 1 shallot, chopped
- 1 vegan pizza dough
- 2 tablespoons parsley /30G
- salt and pepper

Instructions:

1) Preheat mid-air fryer to 400° F or 205°C .
2) Slice the pizza dough into squares. Set aside.
3) Mix the oyster mushroom, shallot, bell pepper and parsley in a mixing bowl.
4) Season with salt and pepper to taste.
5) Place the topping on top of the pizza squares and then place it in the air fryer.
6) Cook for 10 minutes.

Nutrition information:

- Calories per serving: 100
- Carbohydrates: 15.67g

- Protein: 2.9g
- Fat:2.89 g

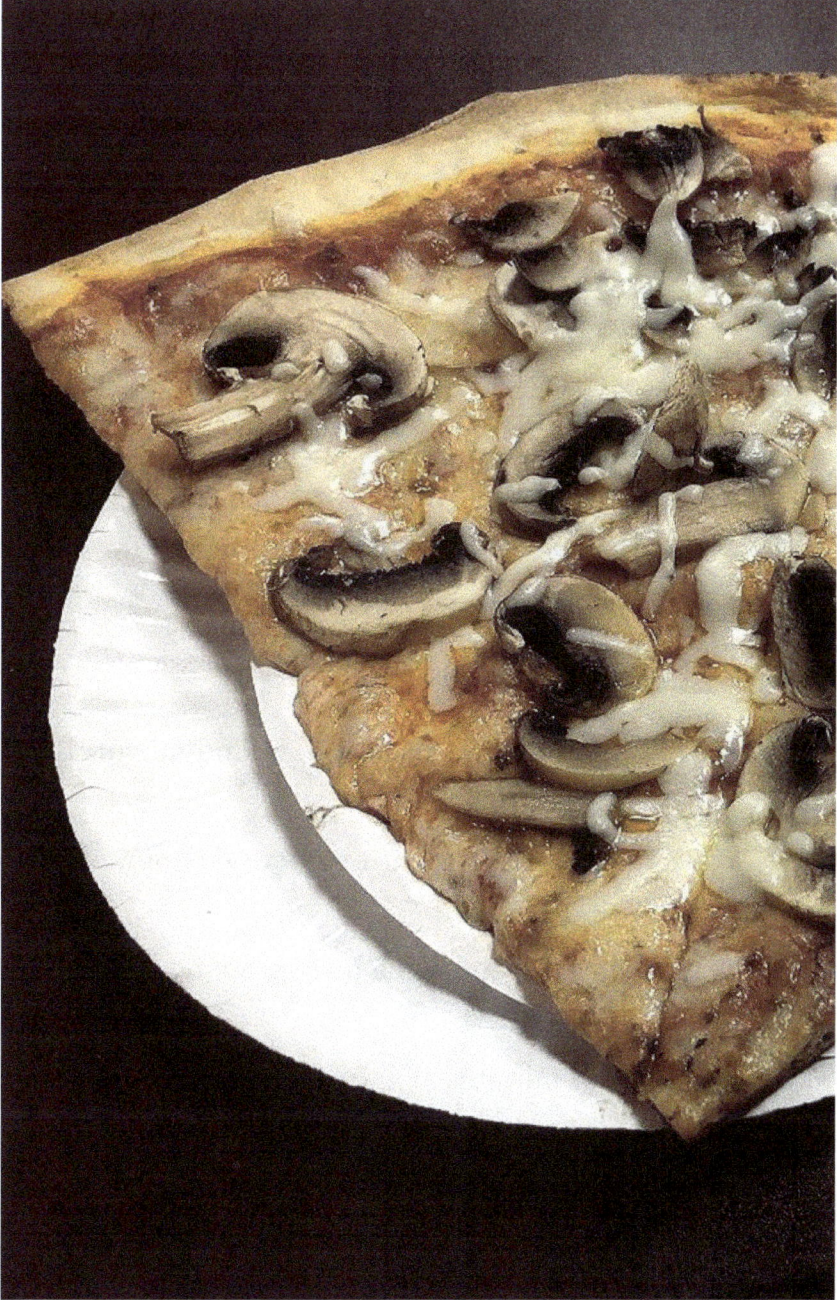

Mushrooms Marinated in Garlic Coco-Aminos

Serves: 8

Cooking Time: 20 minutes

Ingredients:

- ¼ cup coconut aminos /32.5G
- 2 cloves of garlic, minced
- 2 pounds mushrooms, sliced /900G
- 3 tablespoons olive oil /45ML

Instructions:

1) Place all ingredients inside a bowl and mix until well combined.
2) Place in the fridge to marinate for two hours.
3) Preheat the air fryer for 5 minutes.
4) Place the mushrooms in a heat-proof bowl. Place the bowl in the air fryer.
5) Cook for 20 minutes at 350° F or 177°C .

Nutrition information:

- Calories per serving: 467
- Carbohydrates: 86g
- Protein: 6.2g
- Fat: 10.9

Mushrooms Stuffed with Cream Cheese-Pesto

Serves: 5

Cooking Time: 15

Ingredients:

- ¼ cup olive oil /62.5ML
- ½ cup cream cheese /65G
- ½ cup pine nuts /65G
- 1 cup basil leaves /130G
- 1 tablespoon fresh lemon juice, freshly squeezed /15ML
- 1-pound cremini mushrooms stalk removed /450G
- Salt to taste

Instructions

1) Place all ingredients except the mushrooms inside a blender.
2) Blend until smooth.
3) Put some of the mix around the side of the place that the stalks were removed.
4) Place the mushrooms in the fryer basket.
5) Cook for 15minutes at 350° F or 177°C preheated air fryer.

Nutrition information:

- Calories per serving: 585
- Carbohydrates: 71.2g
- Protein; 12,6g
- Fat: 27.8g

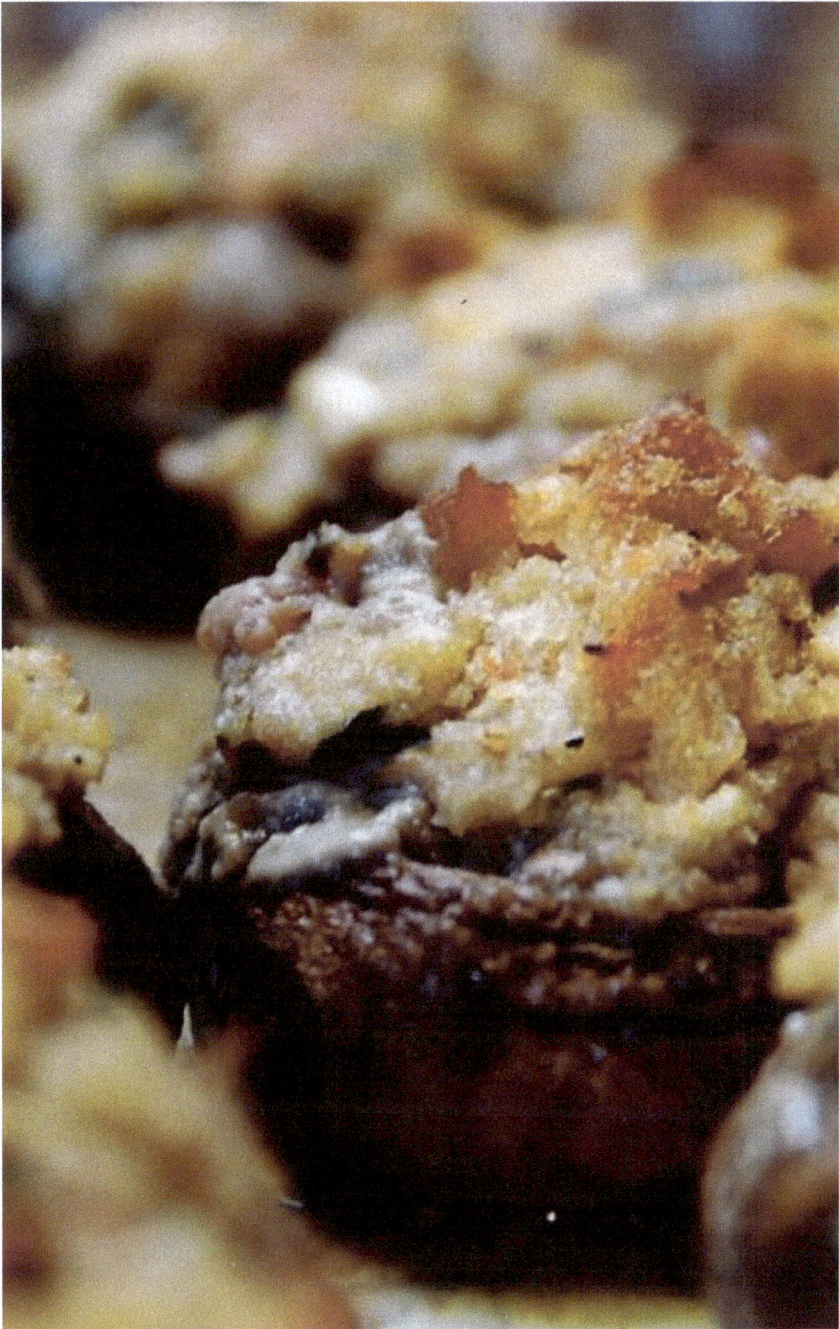

Open-Faced Vegan Flatbread-wich

Serves: 4

Cooking Time: 25 minutes

Ingredients:

- 1 can chickpeas, drained and rinsed
- 1 medium-sized head of cauliflower, cut into florets
- 1 tablespoon extra-virgin essential olive oil /15ML
- 2 ripe avocados, mashed
- 2 tablespoons lemon juice /30ML
- 4 flatbreads, toasted
- salt and pepper to taste

Instructions:

1) Preheat the air fryer to 425° F or 219°C .
2) Add the cauliflower, chickpeas, olive oil, and fresh lemon juice to a mixing bowl. Season with salt and pepper to taste. Mix well.
3) Place inside the air fryer basket and cook for 25 minutes.
4) After cooking, place 50 % of the flatbread and add avocado mash.
5) Season with salt and pepper to taste.
6) Serve with hot sauce.

Nutrition information:

- Calories per serving: 529
- Carbohydrates: 65g
- Protein:11 g
- Fat: 25g

Orange Glazed Fried Tofu

Servings per Recipe: 4

Cooking Time: 25 minutes

Ingredients:

- 1 Tablespoon cornstarch (or arrowroot powder) /15G
- 1 Tablespoon tamari /15G
- 1-pound extra-firm tofu drained and pressed (or use super-firm tofu), cut in cubes /450G

Sauce Ingredients:

- 1 teaspoon orange zest /30G
- 2 teaspoons cornstarch (or arrowroot powder) /10G
- 1 teaspoon fresh ginger minced /5G
- 1 teaspoon fresh garlic minced /5G
- 1 Tablespoon pure maple syrup /15ML
- 1/2 cup water /125ML
- 1/3 cup orange juice /83ML
- 1/4 teaspoon crushed red pepper flakes /1.25G

Instructions:

1) Mix tofu with tamari as well as a tablespoon of cornstarch in a bowl. Marinate for about 15 minutes. Mix well frequently.
2) Mix the sauce ingredients in a bowl and set aside.

3) Grease baking pan of air fryer with cooking spray. Add tofu for 10 Minutes, cook at 390° F or 199°C . Halfway through cooking time, stir. Cook for an additional 10 minutes.

4) Add the sauce, mix well to coat. Cook again for 5 minutes.

5) Serve and enjoy

Nutrition Information:

- Calories per Serving: 63
- Carbs: 11.0g
- Protein: 8.0g
- Fat: 3.0g

Beef Brisket Recipe from Texas

Serves: 8

Cooking Time: one hour and 30 Minutes

Ingredients:

- 1 ½ cup beef stock /375ML
- 1 bay leaf
- 1 tablespoon garlic powder /15G
- 1 tablespoon onion powder /15G
- 2 pounds beef brisket, trimmed /900G
- 2 tablespoons chili powder /30G
- 2 teaspoons dry mustard /10G
- 4 tablespoons organic olive oil /60 ML
- Salt and pepper to taste

Instructions:

1) Preheat the air fryer for 5 minutes.
2) Place all ingredients in the deep baking pan.
3) Bake for an hour and 30 Minutes at 400° F or 205°C .
4) Stir the beef after every 30 minutes to allow the beef to soak in the sauce.

Nutrition information:

- Calories per serving: 306
- Carbohydrates: 3.8g

- Protein: 18.3g
- Fat: 24.1g

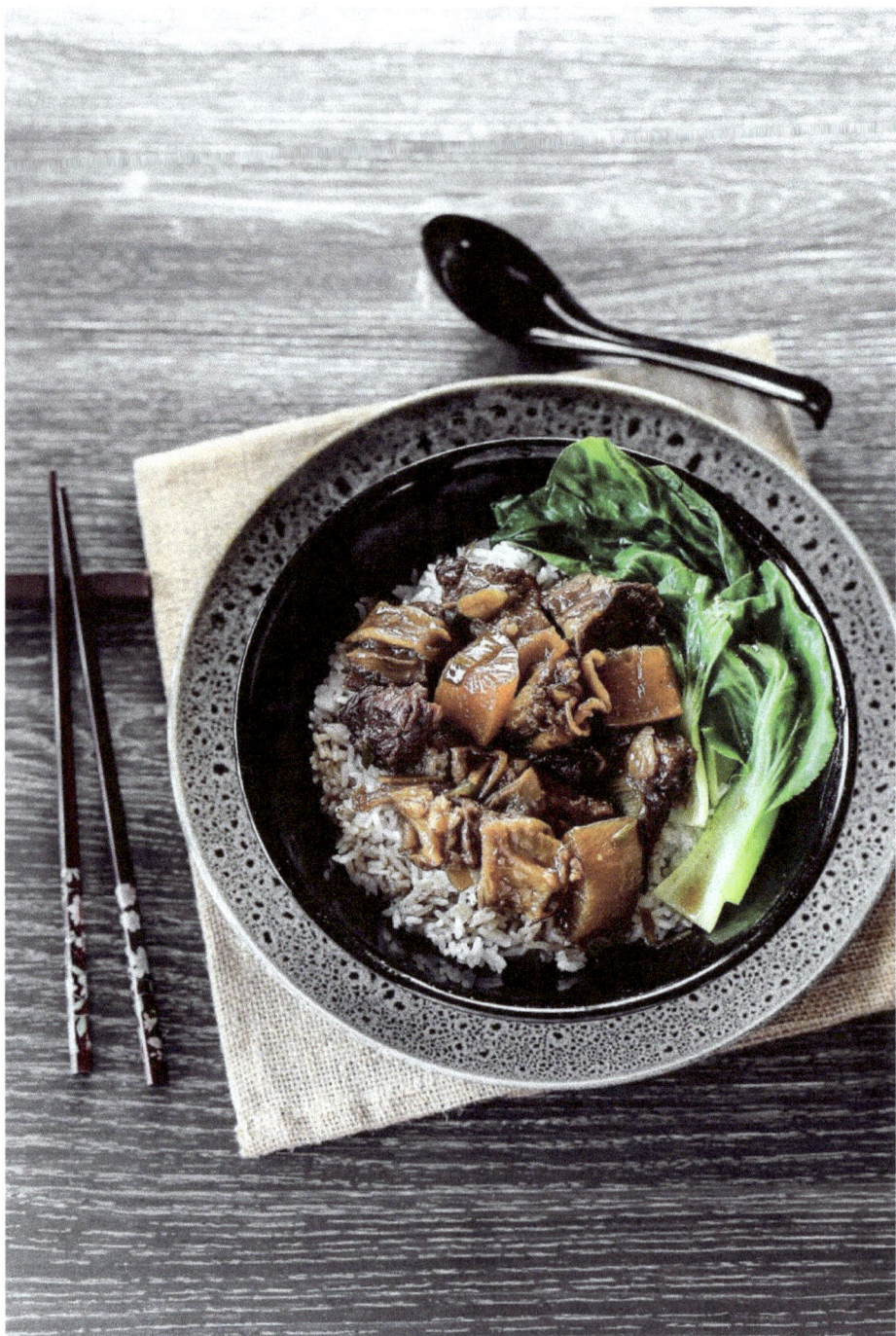

Beef Recipe Texas-Rodeo Style

Servings per Recipe: 6

Cooking Time: an hour

Ingredients:

- ½ cup honey /125ML
- ½ cup ketchup /125ML
- ½ teaspoon dry mustard /2.5G
- 1 clove of garlic, minced
- 1 tablespoon chili powder /15G
- 2 onion, chopped
- 3 pounds beef steak sliced /1350G
- Salt and pepper to taste

Instructions:

1) Place all ingredients in a Ziploc bag, place in the fridge and allow to marinate for about 120 minutes.
2) Preheat mid-air fryer to 390O F or 199°C .
3) Place the grill pan in the air fryer.
4) Grill the beef for 15 minutes per batch, turnover every 8 minutes for even grilling.
5) Meanwhile, pour the marinade over a saucepan and allow it to simmer over medium heat.
6) Baste the beef with sauce before serving.

Nutrition information:

- Calories per serving: 542
- Carbs: 49g
- Protein: 37g
- Fat: 22g

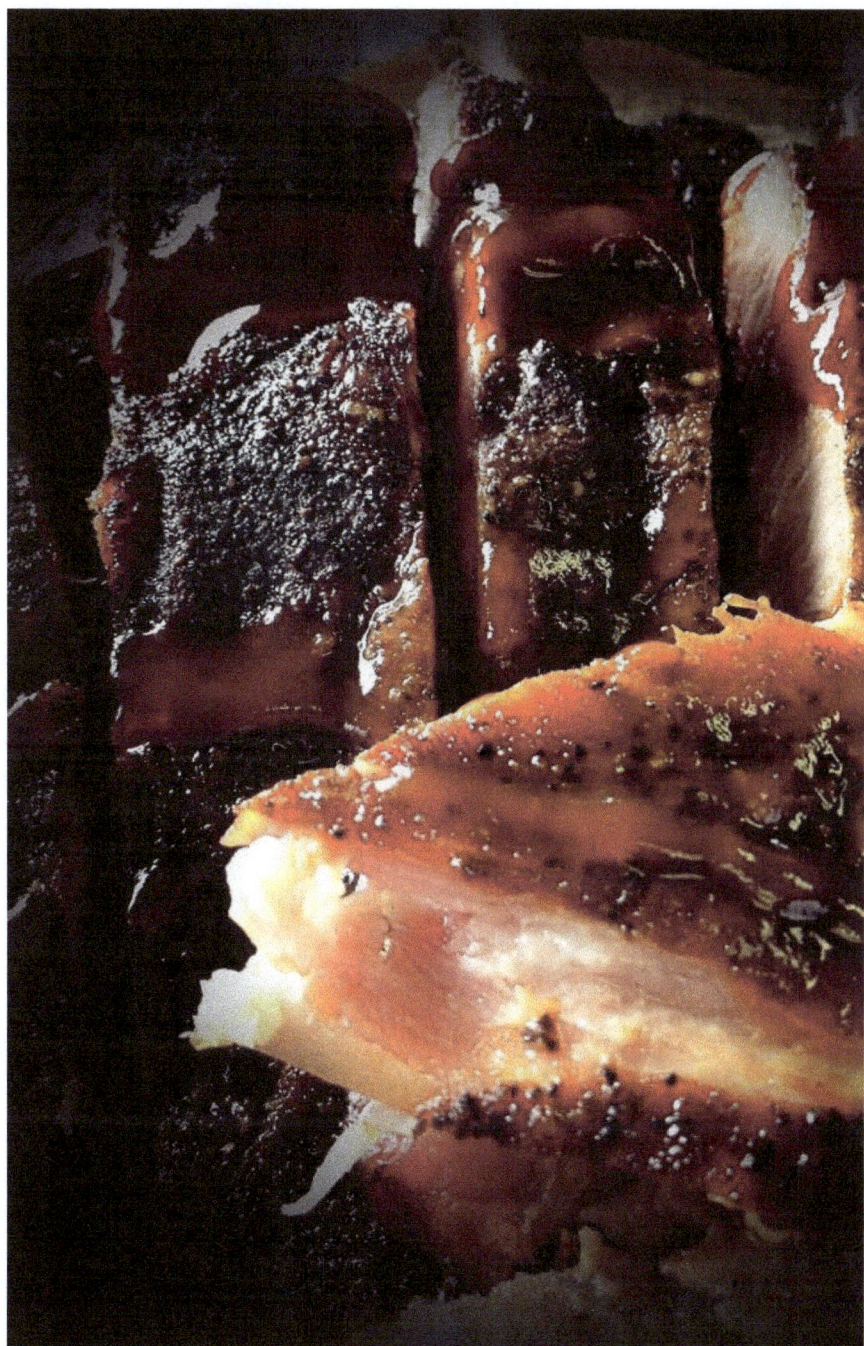

Beef Roast in Worcestershire-Rosemary

Serves: 6

Cooking Time: 2 hours

Ingredients:

- 1 onion, chopped
- 1 tablespoon butter /15G
- 1 tablespoon Worcestershire sauce /15ML
- 1 teaspoon rosemary /5G
- 1 teaspoon thyme /5G
- 1-pound beef chuck roast /450G
- 2 cloves of garlic, minced
- 2 tablespoons olive oil /30ML
- 3 cups water /750ML
- 3 stalks of celery, sliced

Instructions:

1) Preheat the air fryer for 5 minutes.
2) Place all ingredients in a deep baking dish that may fit into a mid-air fryer.
3) Bake for 120 minutes at 350° F or 177°C .
4) Steam the meat using its sauce, stir every 30 minutes until cooked.

Nutrition information:

- Calories per serving: 260
- Carbohydrates: 2.9g
- Protein: 17.5g
- Fat: 19.8

Beefy 'n Cheesy Spanish Rice Casserole

Servings per Recipe: 3

Cooking Time: 50 minutes

Ingredients:

- 2 tablespoons chopped green bell pepper /30G
- 1 tablespoon chopped fresh cilantro /15G
- 1/2-pound lean ground beef /225G
- 1/2 cup water /125ML
- 1/2 teaspoon salt /2.5G
- 1/2 teaspoon brown sugar /2.5G
- 1/2 pinch ground black pepper
- 1/3 cup uncooked long-grain rice /43G
- 1/4 cup finely chopped onion /32.5G
- 1/4 cup chile sauce /62.5ML
- 1/4 teaspoon ground cumin /1.25G
- 1/4 teaspoon Worcestershire sauce /1.25ML
- 1/4 cup shredded Cheddar cheese /32.5G
- 1/2 (14.5 ounces) can canned tomatoes /435G

Instructions:

1) Grease baking pan of air fryer lightly with cooking spray. Add ground beef. Cook on 360° F or 183°C for 10 Minutes. Stir and then crush the beef halfway through cooking time. Remove excess fat.

2) Stir in pepper, Worcestershire sauce, cumin, brown sugar, salt, chile sauce, rice, water, tomatoes, green bell pepper, and onion. Mix well. Cover pan with foil and cook for 25 minutes. Stirring occasionally.

3) Give it one final good stir, press down firmly and sprinkle cheese on top.

4) Do not cover, cook for 15 minutes at 390° F or 199°C until the top is lightly browned.

5) Serve and enjoy with chopped cilantro.

Nutrition Information:

- Calories per Serving: 346
- Carbs: 24.9g
- Protein: 18.5g
- Fat: 19.1g

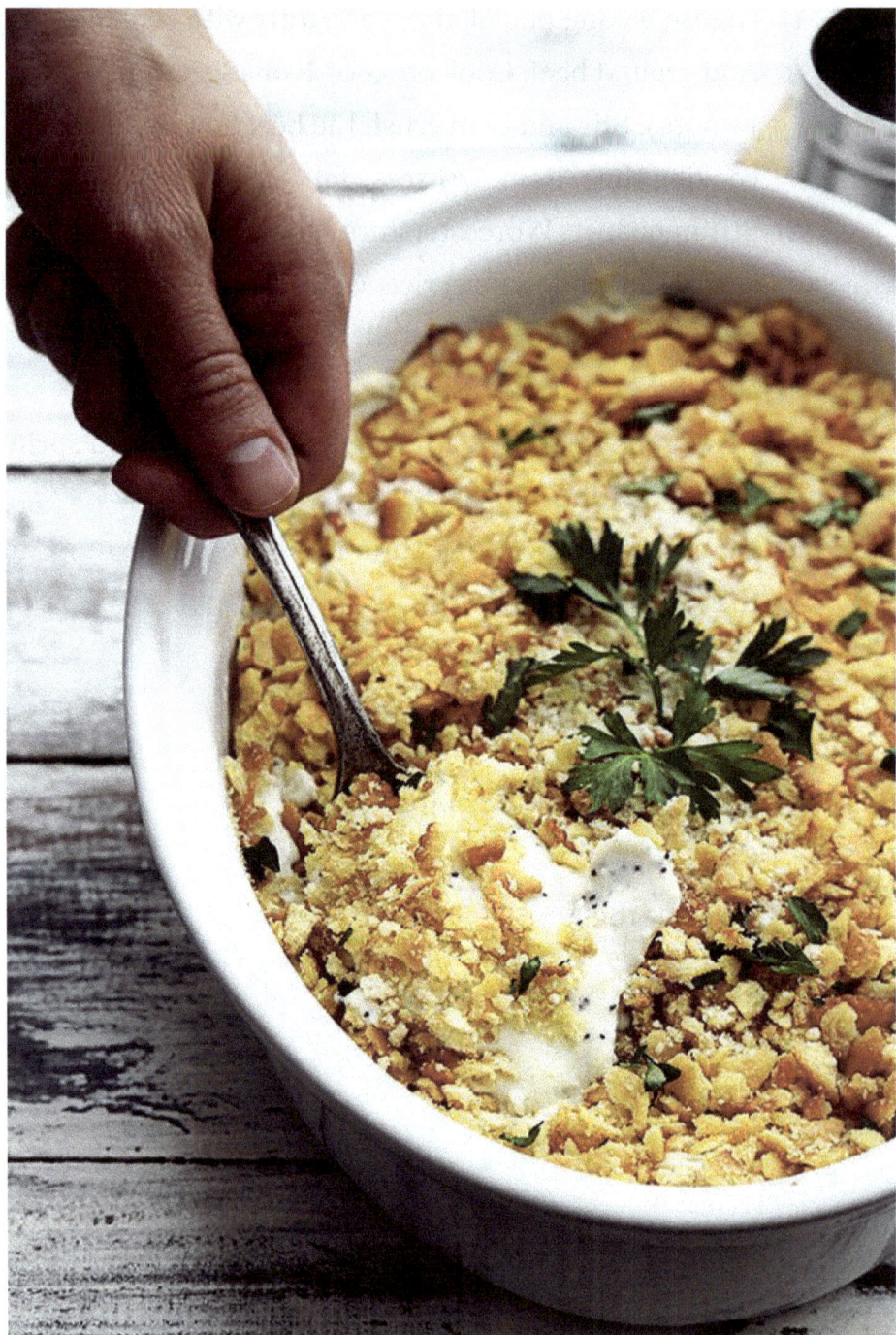

Beefy Bell Pepper 'n Egg Scramble

Servings per Recipe: 4

Cooking Time: 30 Minutes

Ingredients:

- 1 green bell pepper, seeded and chopped
- 1 onion, chopped
- 1-pound ground beef /450G
- 3 cloves of garlic, minced
- 3 tablespoons extra virgin olive oil /45ML
- 6 eggs, beaten
- Salt and pepper to taste

Instructions:

1) Preheat the mid-air fryer for 5 minutes, place a baking pan in it.
2) Mix the bottom beef, onion, garlic, organic olive oil, and bell pepper in a bowl. Season with salt and pepper to taste.
3) Pour inside the beaten eggs and give a good stir.
4) Add the beef to the egg mixture and then place in the air fryer.
5) Bake for 30 minutes at 330° F or 166°C .

Nutrition information:

- Calories per serving: 579
- Carbs: 14.5g
- Protein: 65 8g
- Fat: 28.6g

Ginger-Orange Beef Strips

Servings per Recipe: 3

Cooking Time: 25 minutes

Ingredients:

- 1 ½ pounds stir fry steak slices /675G
- 1 ½ teaspoon sesame oil /7.5ML
- 1 navel oranges, segmented
- 1 tablespoon olive oil /15ML
- 1 tablespoon rice vinegar /15ML
- 1 teaspoon grated ginger /5G
- ·2 scallions, chopped
- 3 cloves of garlic, minced
- 3 tablespoons molasses /45G
- 3 tablespoons soy sauce /22.5ML
- 6 tablespoons cornstarch /90G

Instructions:

1) Preheat mid-air fryer to 330° F or 166°C .
2) Season the steak slices with soy sauce and sprinkle them with cornstarch.
3) Place in the air fryer basket and cook for 25 minutes.
4) Meanwhile, place a pan over medium flame, add oil and allow to warm
5) Sauté the garlic and ginger until wither

6) Stir in the oranges, molasses, and rice vinegar. Season with salt and pepper to taste.

7) Once the meat is cooked, place inside the pan and stir to coat the sauce.

8) Drizzle with sesame oil and garnish with scallions.

Nutrition information:

- Calories per serving: 306
- Carbs: 43.6g
- Protein: 9.4g
- Fat: 10.4g

Gravy Smothered Country Fried Steak

Servings per Recipe: 2

Cooking Time: 25 minutes

Ingredients:

- 1 cup flour /130G
- 1 cup panko bread crumbs /130G
- 1 teaspoon garlic powder /5G
- 1 teaspoon onion powder /5G
- 2 cups milk /500ML
- 2 tablespoons flour /30G
- 3 eggs, beaten
- 6 ounces ground sausage meat /180G
- 6 ounces sirloin steak, pounded thin /180G
- Salt and pepper to taste

Instructions:

1) Preheat mid-air fryer to 330° F or 166°C .
2) Season the steak with salt and pepper to taste.
3) Dip the steak in egg and dredge in flour mixture (consists of flour, bread crumbs, onion powder, and garlic powder).
4) Place in the air fryer and cook for 25 minutes.

5) Meanwhile, place the sausage meat in a saucepan and allow it to release fat. Stir in flour to create a roux and add milk. Season with salt and pepper to taste. Keep stirring before the sauce thickens.

6) Serve the steak with milk gravy

Nutrition information:

- Calories per serving: 1048
- Carbs: 88.1g
- Protein:64.2 g
- Fat: 48.7g

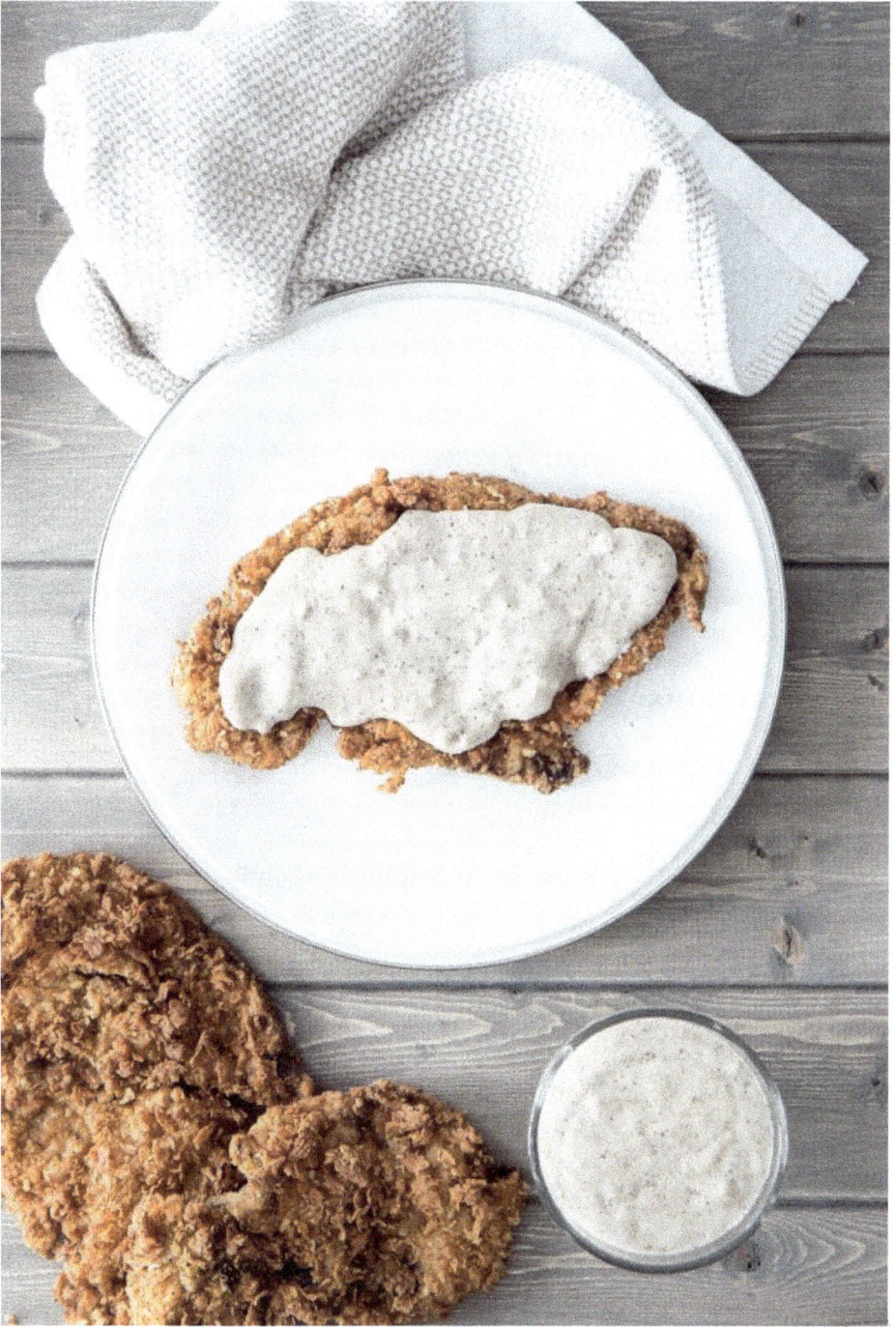

Grilled Beef with Grated Daikon Radish

Servings per Recipe: 2

Cooking Time: 40 minutes

Ingredients:

- ¼ cup grated daikon radish /32.5G
- ½ cup rice wine vinegar /125ML
- ½ cup soy sauce /125ML
- 1 tablespoon olive oil /15ML
- 2 strip steaks
- Salt and pepper to taste

Instructions:

1) Preheat mid-air fryer to 390° F or 199°C .
2) Place the grill pan in the air fryer.
3) Season the steak with salt and pepper.
4) Brush with oil.
5) Grill for 20 Minutes per piece and turn the beef after 10 minutes.
6) Prepare the dipping sauce by combining the soy sauce and vinegar.
7) Serve the steak using the sauce and daikon radish.

Nutrition information:

- Calories per serving: 510

- Carbs:19.3 g
- Protein: 54g
- Fat: 24g

Grilled Prosciutto-Wrapped Fig

Servings per Recipe: 2

Cooking Time: 8 minutes

Ingredients:

- 2 whole figs, sliced in quarters
- 8 prosciutto slices
- Pepper and salt to taste

Instructions:

1) Wrap a prosciutto slice around one slice of fid after which thread into the skewer. Repeat until all ingredients are used. Place on the skewer rack in the air fryer.
2) Cook at 390° F or 199°C for 8 minutes. cook. Turnover skewer after 4 minutes.
3) Serve and enjoy.

Nutrition Information:

- Calories per Serving: 277
- Carbs: 10.7g
- Protein: 36.0g
- Fat: 10.0g

Grilled Sausages with BBQ Sauce

Servings per Recipe: 3

Cooking Time: 30 Minutes

Ingredients:

- ½ cup prepared BBQ sauce /125ML
- 6 sausage links

for Cooking:

1) Preheat the air fryer to 390° F or 199°C .
2) Place the grill pan in the air fryer.
3) Place the sausage links and grill for 30 Minutes.
4) Flip halfway through the cooking time.
5) Before serving brush with prepared BBQ sauce.

Nutrition information:

- Calories per serving: 265
- Carbs: 6.4g
- Protein: 27.7g
- Fat: 14.2g

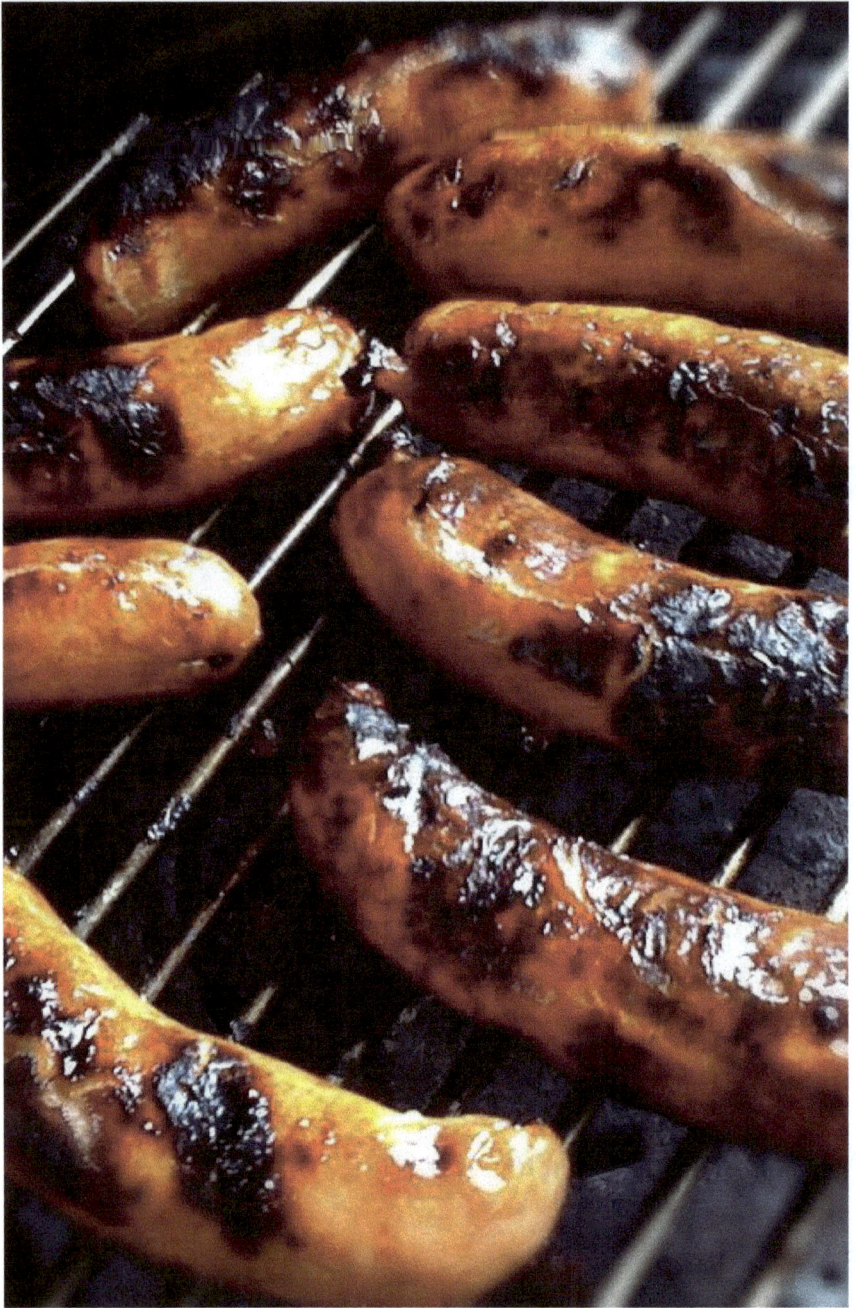

Salted 'n Peppered Scored Beef Chuck

Servings per Recipe: 6

Cooking Time: 1 hour and 30 Minutes

Ingredients:

- 2 ounces black peppercorns /60G
- 2 tablespoons organic olive oil /30ML
- 3 pounds beef chuck roll, scored with a knife /1350G
- 3 tablespoons salt /45G

Instructions:

1) Preheat the air fryer to 390° F or 199°C .
2) Place the grill pan accessory in the air fryer.
3) Season the beef chuck roll with black peppercorns and salt.
4) Brush with organic olive oil and cover top with foil.
5) Grill for 90 minutes
6) Flip the beef every 30 Minutes until evenly cooked.

Nutrition information:

- Calories per serving: 360
- Carbs: 1.4g
- Protein: 46.7g
- Fat: 18g

Salted Corned Beef with Onions

Serves: 12

Cooking Time: 50 minutes

Ingredients:

- 1 large onion, chopped
- 2 tablespoons Dijon mustard /30G
- 3 pounds corned beef brisket, cut into chunks /1350G
- 4 cups water /1Liter
- Salt and pepper to taste

Instructions:

1) Preheat mid-air fryer for 5 minutes
2) Place all ingredients in the baking pan.
3) Cook for 50 minutes at 400° F or 205°C .

Nutrition information:

- Calories per serving: 241
- Carbohydrates: 1.5g
- Protein: 15.2g
- Fat:19.3g

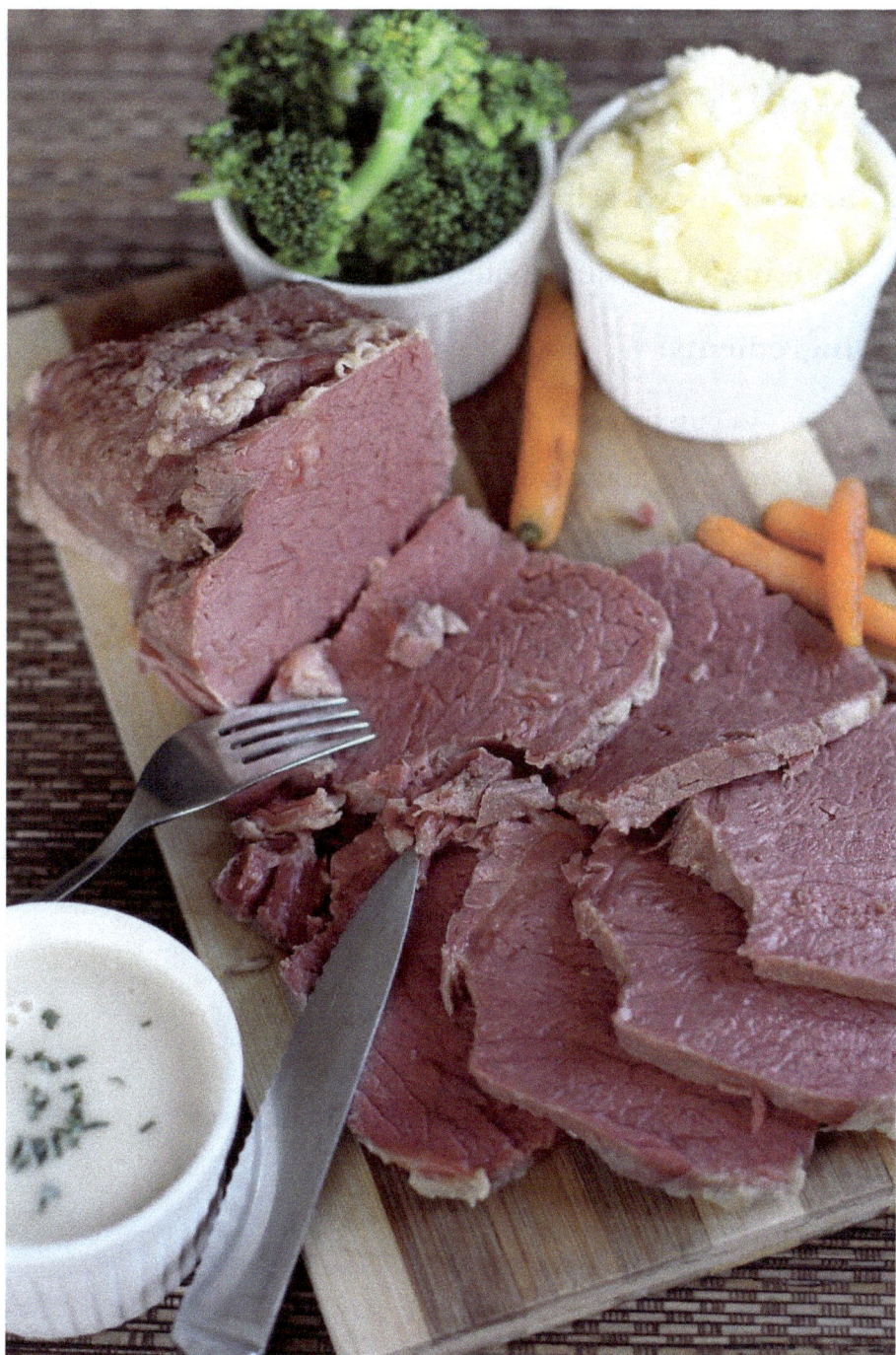

Salted Porterhouse with Sage 'n Thyme Medley

Servings per Recipe: 2

Cooking Time: 40 minutes

Ingredients:

- ¼ cup fish sauce /62.5ML
- 2 porterhouse steaks
- 2 tablespoons marjoram /30G
- 2 tablespoons sage /30G
- 2 tablespoons thyme /30G
- Salt and pepper to taste

Instructions:

1) Place all ingredients in a Ziploc bag, place in the fridge and allow to marinate for 2 hours.
2) Preheat the air fryer to 390° F or 199°C .
3) Place the grill pan accessory in the air fryer.
4) Grill for 20 Minutes per batch.
5) Flip every 10 to give a uniform doneness

Nutrition information:

- Calories per serving: 1189
- Carbs: 6.3g
- Protein: 112.5g

- Fat: 79.3g

Salted Steak Pan-Fried Steak

Serves: 1

Cooking Time: 15

Ingredients:

- 1-pound beef steak, bones removed /450G
- 3 tablespoons coconut oil /45ML
- A dash of oregano
- Salt and pepper to taste

Instructions:

1) Place all ingredients inside a Ziploc bag, place in a fridge and allow to marinate for few hours.
2) Preheat the air fryer.
3) Place the steak in the air fryer and cook for 15 minutes at 400° F or 205°C .

Nutrition information:

- Calories per serving: 1151
- Carbohydrates: 4.2g
- Protein: 65.9g
- Fat: 96.7g

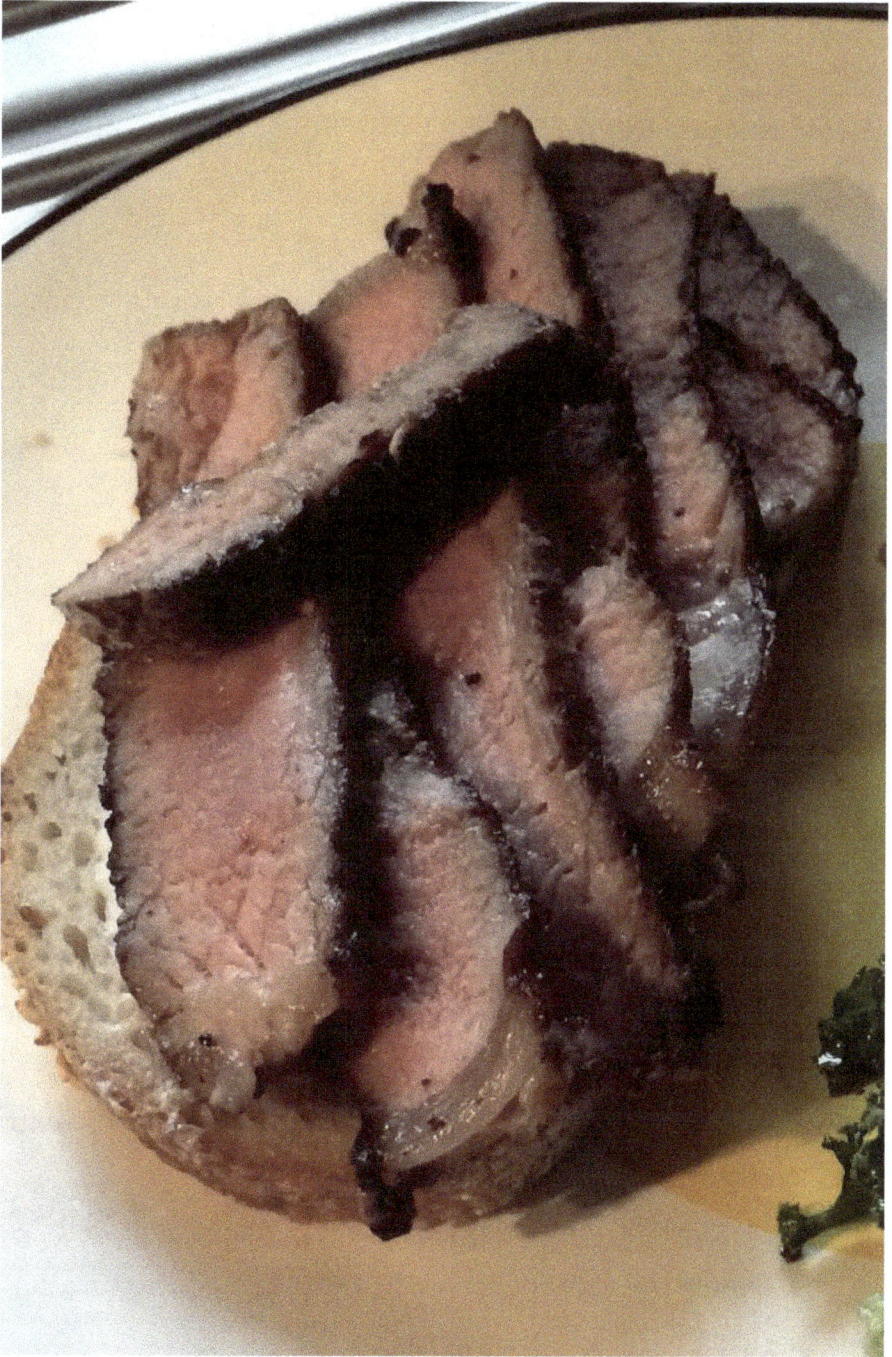

Sausage 'n Cauliflower Frittata

Servings per Recipe: 3

Cooking Time: 27 minutes

Ingredients:

- 1-pound hot pork sausage, diced /450G
- ½ cup shredded Cheddar cheese /65G
- 1 teaspoons salt /5G
- ½ cup milk /125ML
- 1 small cauliflower, riced
- 3 large eggs
- 1/2 (30 ounces) package frozen hash brown potatoes, thawed /900G
- 1/2 teaspoon ground black pepper /2.5G

Instructions:

1) Grease baking pan of air fryer lightly with cooking spray. And add diced sausage and cook for 10 minutes at 360° F or 177°C .

2) Add hash brown and riced cauliflower. Cook extra 5 minutes.

3) Meanwhile, whisk eggs, salt, pepper, and milk well.

4) Evenly spread cheese and pour the egg mixture on the rice.

5) Cook for an additional 12 minutes or until set

6) Serve and revel in.

Nutrition Information:

- Calories per Serving: 612
- Carbs: 33.4g
- Protein: 49.2g
- Fat: 44.6g

Chicken BBQ Recipe from Italy

Servings per Recipe: 2

Cooking Time: 40 minutes

Ingredients

- 1 tablespoon fresh Italian parsley /15G
- 1 tablespoon minced garlic /15G
- 1-pound boneless chicken breasts /450G
- 2 tablespoons tomato paste /30ML
- Salt and pepper to taste

Instructions:

1) Add all ingredients except for the corn in a Ziploc bag. Allow to marinate inside the fridge for a couple of hours.
2) Preheat the air fryer to 390° F or 199°C .
3) Place the grill pan accessory inside the air fryer.
4) Grill the chicken for 40 minutes.

Nutrition information:

- Calories per serving: 292
- Carbs: 6.6g
- Protein: 52.6g
- Fat: 6.1g

Chicken BBQ Recipe from Peru

Servings per Recipe: 4

Cooking Time: 40 minutes

Ingredients:

- ½ teaspoon dried oregano /2.5G
- 1 teaspoon paprika /5G
- 1/3 cup soy sauce /83ML
- 2 ½ pounds chicken, quartered /1125G
- 2 tablespoons fresh lime juice /30ML
- 2 teaspoons ground cumin /10G
- 5 cloves of garlic, minced

Instructions:

1) Add all ingredients in a Ziploc bag and shake to combine everything.
2) Place in a fridge and allow to marinate for few hours.
3) Preheat mid-air fryer to 390° F or 199°C .
4) Place the grill pan accessory inside the air fryer.
5) Grill the chicken for 40 minutes. Flip the chicken every 10 minutes for even grilling.

Nutrition information:

- Calories per serving: 377
- Carbs: 7.9g

- Protein: 59.7g
- Fat: 11.8g

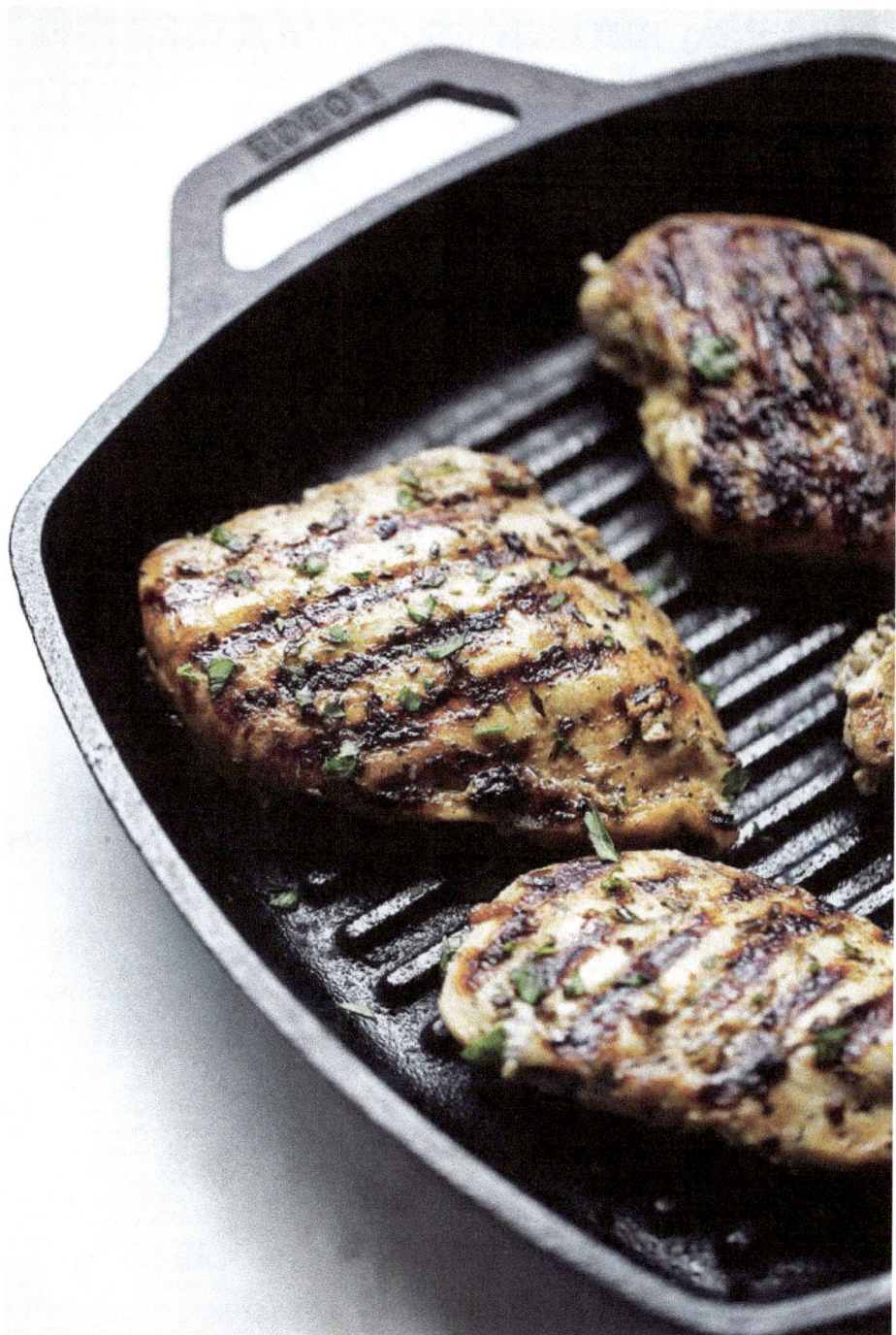

Chicken BBQ with Sweet 'n Sour Sauce

Servings per Recipe: 6

Cooking Time: 40 minutes

Ingredients:

- ¼ cup minced garlic /32.5G
- ¼ cup tomato paste /32.5G
- ¾ cup minced onion /98G
- ¾ cup sugar 98G
- 1 cup soy sauce /250ML
- 1 cup water 250ML
- 1 cup white vinegar 250ML
- 6 chicken drumsticks
- Salt and pepper to taste

Instructions:

1) Place all Ingredients in the Ziploc bag
2) Place the Ziploc bag in a fridge and allow to marinate for 120 minutes.
3) Preheat the air fryer to 390° F or 199°C .
4) Place the grill pan accessory in the air fryer.
5) Grill the chicken for 40 minutes.
6) Flip the chicken every 10 minutes for only grilling.
7) Meanwhile, pour the marinade in a saucepan, place on a medium-flame and allow to warm till the sauce thickens.

8) Brush the chicken lavishly with sauce. Serve and enjoy.

Nutrition information:

- Calories per serving: 407
- Carbs:29.6 g
- Protein: 27.8g
- Fat: 19.7g

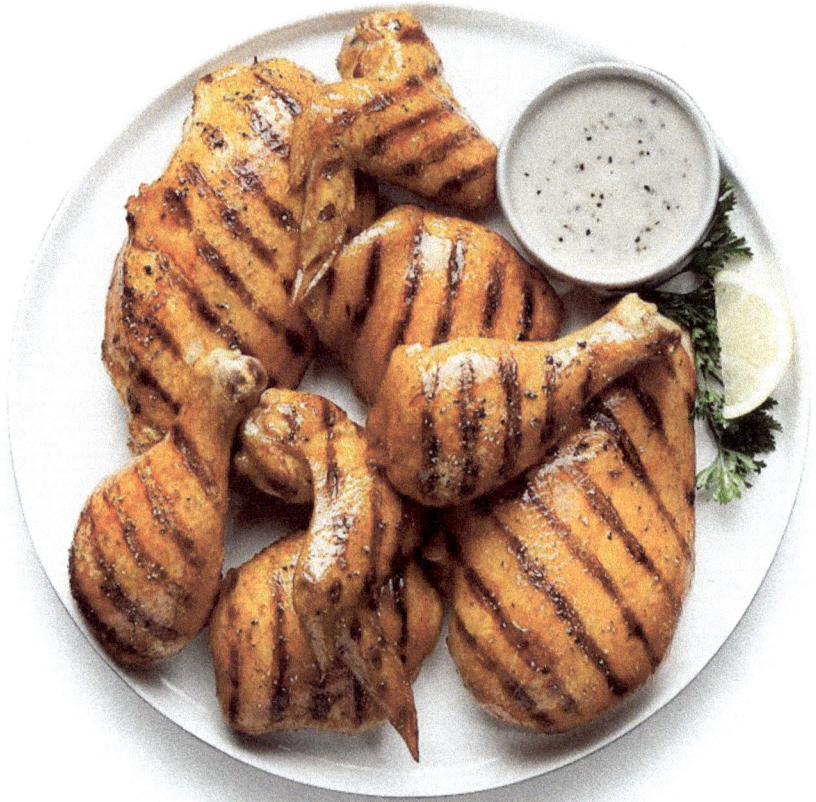

Chicken Fry Recipe in the Mediterranean

Servings per Recipe: 2

Cooking Time: 21 minutes

Ingredients:

- 2 boneless skinless chicken white meat halves (6 ounces or 180G each)
- 3 tablespoons organic olive oil /45ML
- 6 pitted Greek or ripe olives, sliced
- 2 tablespoons capers, drained /30G
- 1/2-pint grape tomatoes
- 1/4 teaspoon salt /1.25G
- 1/4 teaspoon pepper /1.25G

Instructions:

1) Grease a pan lightly with oil.

2) Add chicken and season with pepper and salt to taste.

3) Preheat air fryer at 390O F or 199°C . Place chicken in the air fryer, allow each side to Brown for 3 minutes.

4) Add capers, olives, tomatoes, and oil. Mix well.

5) Cook for 15 minutes, cook at 330O F or 166°C .

6) Serve and enjoy

Nutrition Information:

- Calories per Serving: 330
- Carbs: 6.0g
- Protein: 36.0g
- Fat: 18.0g

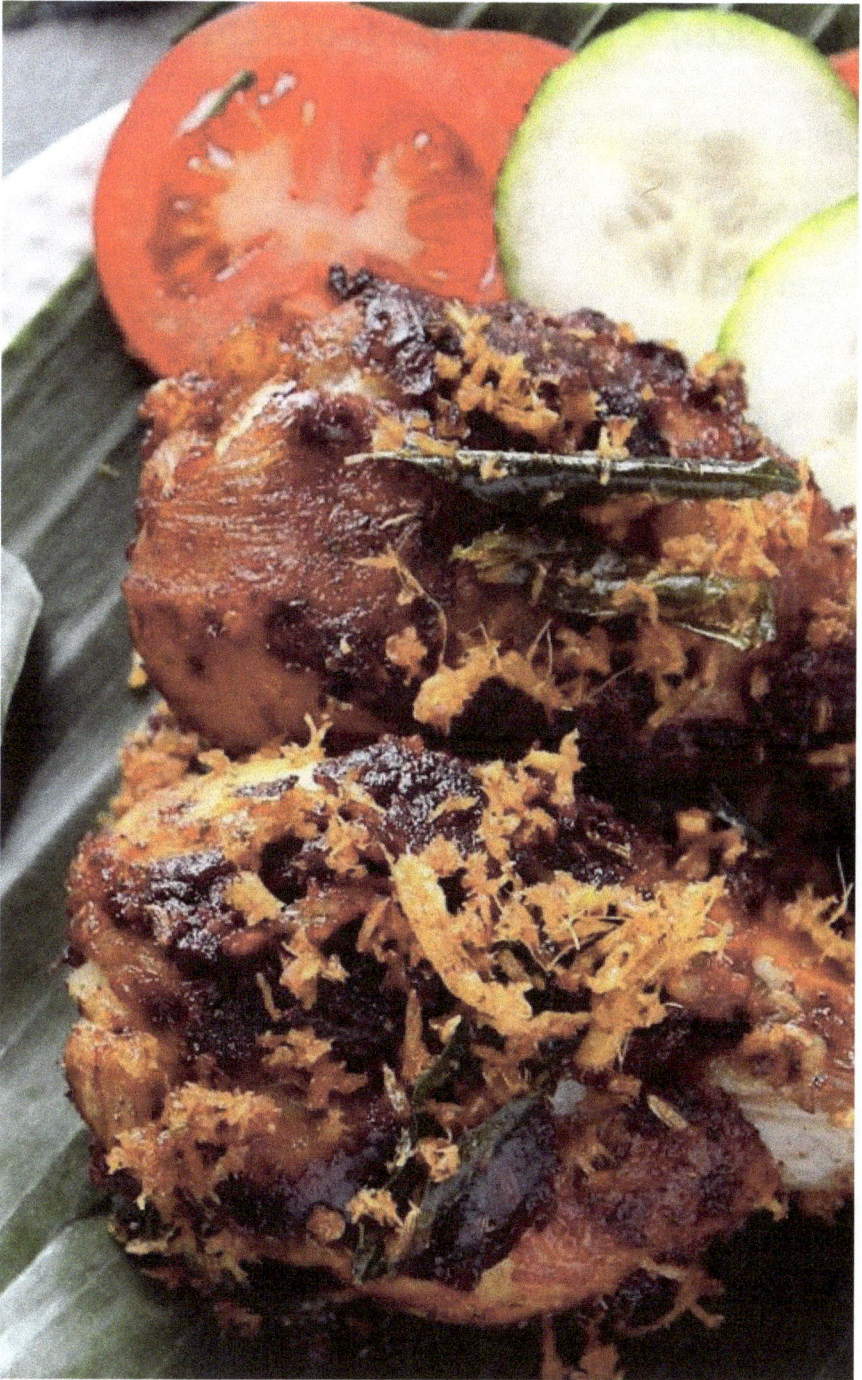

Chicken Grill Recipe from California

Servings per Recipe: 4

Cooking Time: 40 minutes

Ingredients:

- ¾ cup balsamic vinegar /188ML
- 1 teaspoon garlic powder /5G
- 2 tablespoons extra virgin organic olive oil /30ML
- 2 tablespoons honey /30ML
- 2 teaspoons Italian seasoning /10G
- 4 boneless chicken breasts
- 4 slices mozzarella
- 4 slices of avocado
- 4 slices of tomato
- Balsamic vinegar for drizzling
- Salt and pepper to taste

Instructions:

1) Mix the balsamic vinegar, garlic powder, honey, organic olive oil, Italian seasoning, salt, pepper, and chicken in a Ziploc bag. Allow to marinate in the fridge for about 2 hours.

2) Preheat air fryer to 390° F or 199°C .

3) Place the grill pan accessory in the air fryer.

4) Put the chicken on the grill and cook for 40 minutes.

5) Flip the chicken every 10 Minutes to grill evenly.

6) Serve the chicken with mozzarella, avocado, and tomato. Drizzle with balsamic vinegar.

Nutrition information:

- Calories per serving: 853
- Carbs: 43.2g
- Protein:69.4 g
- Fat: 44.7g

Garlic Paprika Rubbed Chicken Breasts

Serves: 4

Cooking Time: 30 Minutes

Ingredients:

- 1 tablespoon stevia powder /15G
- 2 tablespoons fresh lemon juice, freshly squeezed /30ML
- 2 tablespoons Spanish paprika /30G
- 2 teaspoons minced garlic /10G
- 3 tablespoons extra virgin olive oil /45ML
- 4 boneless chicken breasts
- Salt and pepper to taste

Instructions:

1) Preheat the air fryer for 5 minutes.
2) Place all ingredients inside a baking dish. Stir to mix.
3) Place the chicken pieces in the air fryer.
4) Cook for 30 minutes at 325° F or 163°C .

Nutrition information:

- Calories per serving:424
- Carbohydrates: 3.9g
- Protein: 62.2g
- Fat: 17.7g

Garlic Rosemary Roasted Chicken

Serves: 6

Cooking Time: 50 minutes

Ingredients:

- 1 tsp rosemary /5G
- 2 pounds whole chicken /900G
- 4 cloves of garlic, minced
- Salt and pepper to taste

Instructions:

1) Season the whole chicken well with garlic, salt, and pepper.
2) Place inside air fryer basket.
3) Cook for 30 Minutes at 330° F or 166°C .
4) Flip the chicken and cook for another 20 minutes.

Nutrition information:

- Calories per serving: 328
- Carbohydrates: 30.8g
- Protein: 14.5g
- Fat: 16.3g

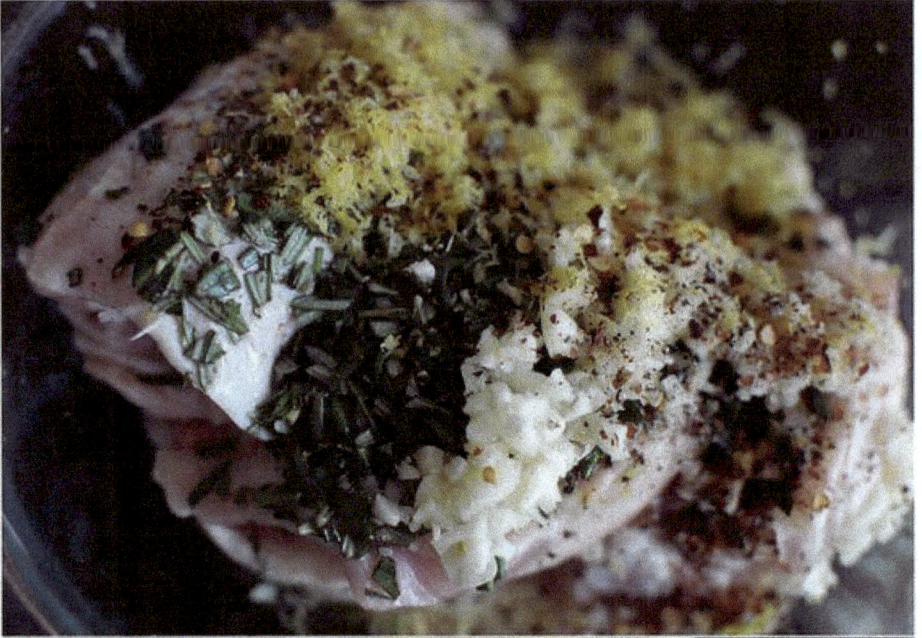

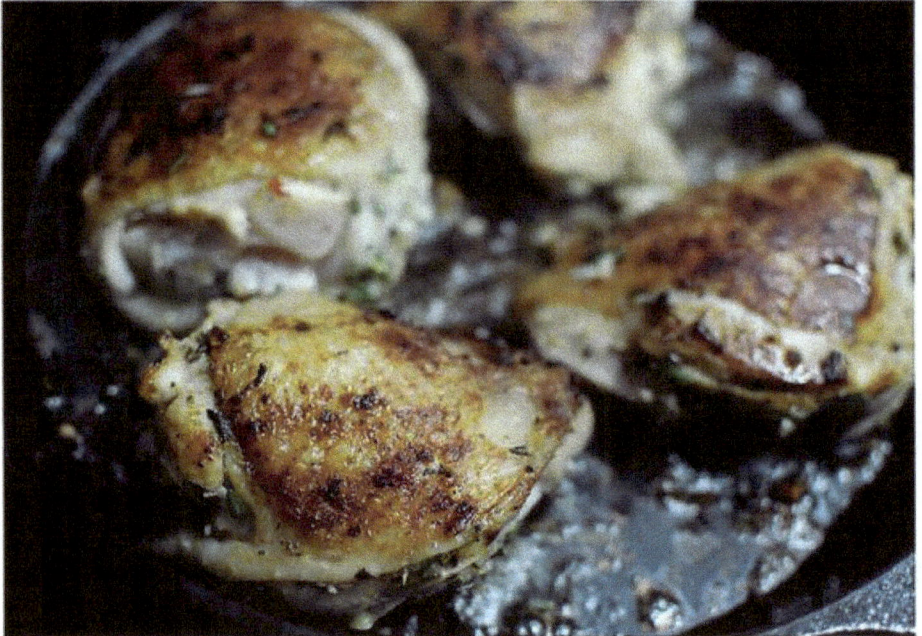

Ginger Garam Masala Rubbed Chicken

Serves: 4

Cooking Time: 50 minutes

Ingredients:

- 1 bell pepper, seeded and julienned
- 1 cup coconut milk /250ML
- 1 teaspoon coriander powder /5G
- 1 teaspoon garam masala /5G
- 1 teaspoon turmeric powder /5G
- 1 thumb-size ginger, grated
- 1 whole chicken, sliced into
- 2 tablespoons essential olive oil /30ML

Instructions:

1) Preheat mid-air fryer for 5 minutes.
2) Place all ingredients in the baking dish.
3) Stir to combine completely.
4) Place inside the air fryer.
5) Cook for 50 minutes at 350° F or 177°C .

Nutrition information:

- Calories per serving: 699
- Carbohydrates: 4.9g
- Protein: 44.5g

- Fat: 55.7g

Greens 'n Turkey sausage Frittata

Servings per Recipe: 2

Cooking Time: 20 Minutes

Ingredients:

- ½ cup cheddar cheese finely grated, extra sharp /65G
- ½ cup milk skimmed /125ML
- 1/2-pound breakfast turkey sausage /225G
- 1/4 tsp cayenne /1.25G
- 1/4 tsp garlic powder /1.25G
- 2-oz hash browns frozen, shredded /60G
- 3 eggs
- 5-oz pre-cut mixed greens (kale, spinach, swiss chard or other things that are you will find) /150G
- green onions for serving
- salt to taste

Instructions:

1) Lightly oil the baking pan of the air fryer with cooking spray and add turkey sausage.
2) For 5 minutes, cook on 360° F or 183°C . Cut the sausage in half.
3) Whisk eggs in a bowl. Season with salt, cayenne, and garlic powder. Add milk and whisk well.

4) Remove the basket and cut more sausage. Stir in frozen hash brown and continue cooking for 5 minutes.

5) Toss in mixed greens and cheese.

6) Pour egg mixture over hash brown mixture.

7) Cook for an additional 10 minutes until eggs are cooked.

8) Sprinkle green onions and let it sit for a minute.

9) Serve and enjoy.

Nutrition Information:

- Calories per Serving: 616
- Carbs: 39.8g
- Protein: 39.7g
- Fat: 33.1g

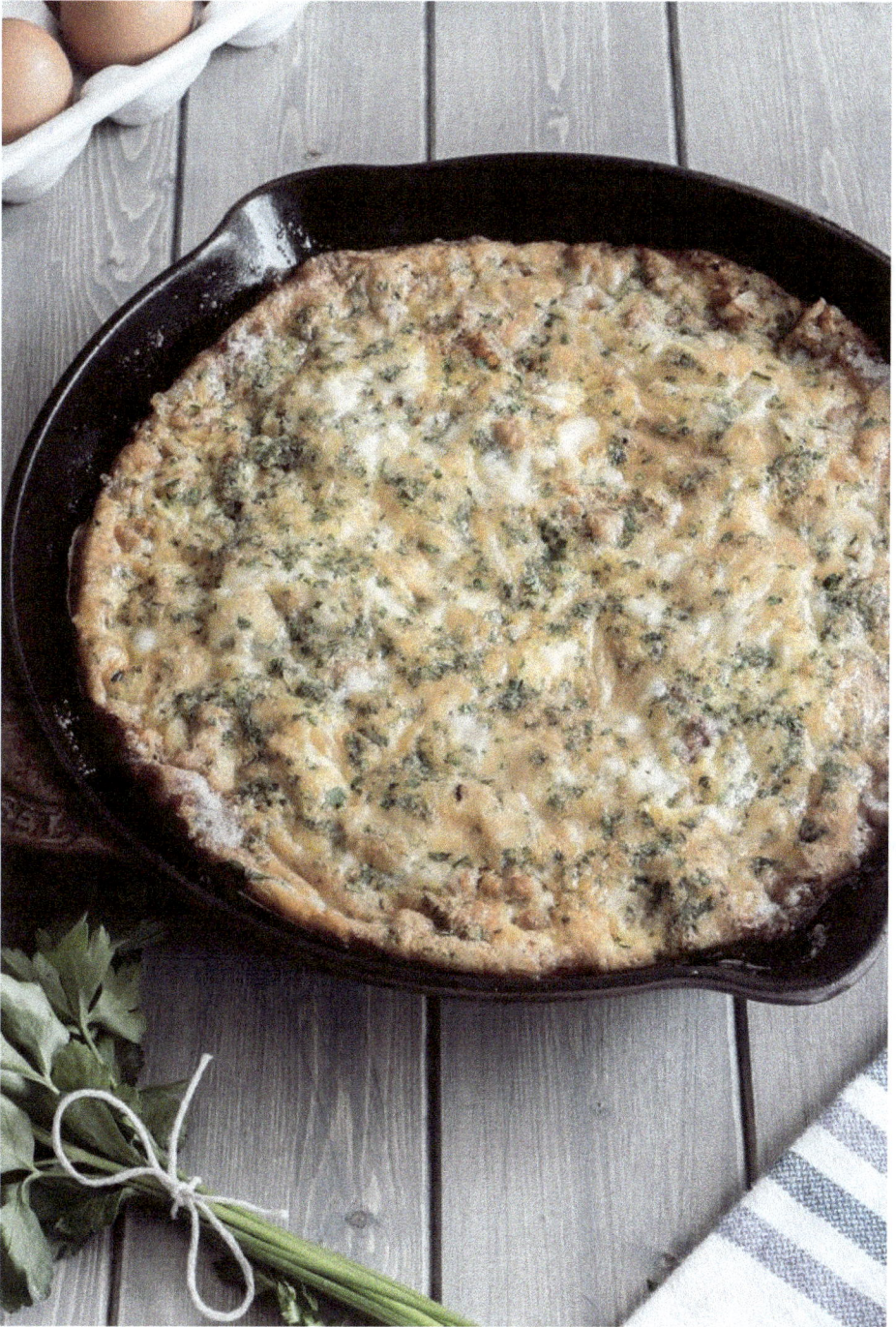

www.ingramcontent.com/pod-product-compliance
Lightning Source LLC
Chambersburg PA
CBHW050746030426
42336CB00012B/1676